# GETTING PREGNANT

## A Guide for the Infertile Couple

### DR. DEREK LLEWELLYN-JONES

**Delta**

A Delta Book
Published by
Dell Publishing
a division of
Bantam Doubleday Dell Publishing Group, Inc.
666 Fifth Avenue
New York, New York 10103

This work was first published in Australia by Ashwood House Medical.

Library of Congress Cataloging-in-Publication Data

Llewellyn-Jones, Derek
    Getting pregnant : a guide for the infertile couple / Derek
Llewellyn-Jones.
    p.    cm.
Includes bibliographical references (p.    ) and index.
ISBN 0-385-30424-2
1. Infertility—Popular works. I. Title.
RC889.L59 1991
616.6'92—dc20

Manufactured in the United States of America
Published simultaneously in Canada
First U.S.A. printing — July 1991

Edited by Marjorie Pressley
Illustrations by Julia McLeish
10 9 8 7 6 5 4 3 2 1
RRH

# Contents

# Introduction —
# Why This Book Was Written

This book was written because of the relatively large numbers of couples who are involuntarily childless. The numbers are impressive, if disconcerting. It has been estimated that one couple in every 7 has not conceived within 1 year of trying and can be considered infertile. When this cold statistic is translated into numbers of couples, over 3 million couples in Canada and the United States of America, over 400 000 couples in Britain and over 100 000 couples in Australia and New Zealand are infertile. This can be put another way. About 3½ million marriages take place in the countries mentioned each year. If 14 per cent of couples are involuntarily infertile, at least 400 000 couples may seek advice about investigation and treatment each year.

It is also known that the proportion of infertile couples increases with the age of the woman and the duration of the marriage. When the woman is under the age of 25, one couple in 15 is infertile; when the woman is aged between 25 and 34, the proportion increases to one in 10 and when the woman is aged between 40 and 49 to eight of every 10.

Infertility is not a woman's problem but a couple's problem — that is why this book has been written. It was also written for family doctors, who are generally the first contact the couple make when seeking help for their infertility problem. Many doctors have a limited knowledge about infertility and, because of the congestion of the medical course, may have listened to a single lecture and attended an infertility clinic only once before entering practice.

It may seem ambitious to write a book for family doctors and for their infertile patients, but I believe that it is not. Most infertile couples read widely (if not wisely) about their problem, and it would be condescending to "write down" to them. But as some may not be overfamiliar with medical terms, I have added a glossary.

Infertility is encompassed by an astonishing amount of mystery and many proposed investigations and treatments are based more on magic than medicine. Magic has long played a part in helping barren women. It was needed, when no other treatment was available, to help a childless woman avoid rejection by her husband and by her community. This rejection is emphasized by Ruth's anguished cry "Give me children or else I die." Fertility rites were (and are) commonplace in many societies. Ceremonials, rituals, invocations, contact with fertility symbols, prayers, diets, sexual positions and meditation have been used by women to try to cure their infertility. And some women have become pregnant following the magical procedure. For this reason it is not surprising that modern medicine also adopts procedures that have a magical basis!

When the mystery and the magic of the investigations and treatment of infertility are peeled away, it becomes apparent that the couple need to answer certain questions and that certain tests are required to establish the cause of their infertility as far as is possible. As in most medical matters, the investigations start when the doctor meets with the woman (and her partner) and they talk. The purpose of this interview is to obtain a good medical history, so that the doctor may ascertain the person's feelings and select the tests he thinks are most appropriate. Each member of an infertile couple has responsibilities in this interview. Unless he or she is prepared to answer all the questions honestly and completely some of the tests chosen may not be appropriate. As some of the questions are about sensitive matters, for example frequency of sexual intercourse, previous induced abortions and sexually transmitted diseases, it is understandable that the person may be reluctant to answer honestly. It is important that this reluctance is overcome and that each partner feels he or she can speak freely knowing that what is said will remain confidential.

Such questions and the tests required often put the couple under stress. It is likely that they are already under stress, perhaps from over-anxious parents who wish to become grandparents, or from observing some of their friends who seem to achieve a pregnancy effortlessly.

The failure to become pregnant may induce a feeling of unworthiness and a reduction in the self-esteem of the woman. After all, society and family *expect* a couple to have children and in some groups childbirth is seen as a sign of adulthood and maturity. Couples may also feel vulnerable during the course of infertility investigations. Both partners may feel that they are no longer in control of their bodies, the control having passed to the doctor. Many of the tests require an invasion of a particularly intimate area of the body, with no certainty that the tests will prove to be helpful or even informative. In these circumstances, either partner, but more often the woman, may develop feelings of anger or guilt, which alternate with depression or grief. The marital relationship of the couple may suffer because of the stress. More particularly, their sexual relationship may cease to be a mutually intimately enjoyed pleasure and may become a coldy clinical act, as yet another attempt is made to achieve a pregnancy.

In the face of these stresses it is important that the couple have a sensitive, empathetic, knowledgeable doctor, whom they can trust. They need a doctor who is prepared to and is able to communicate with the couple. An explanation of what is proposed and why the test is necessary will reduce the anxiety considerably. In some cases the family doctor carries out all the basic tests and, when necessary, refers the couple to an appropriate specialist (a gynecologist, an endocrinologist or an andrologist). In other instances the couple ask to be referred to an infertility clinic (which is usually staffed by, or has access to, several specialists), or to a doctor who has made infertility his or her speciality.

The book is written in the hope that infertile couples and their doctors will be helped in their joint pursuit — to help the couple have a baby.

# 1
## The Infertile Couple

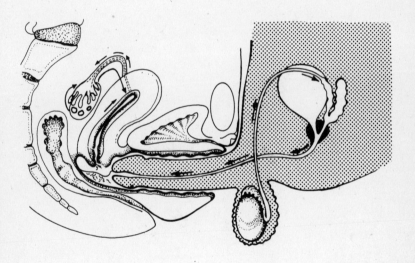

# 1

# The Infertile Couple

Despite increased sexual experimentation, and new life-styles, despite the fact that increasing career opportunities have occurred in recent years, over 85 per cent of women want to bear and nurture a child, and a similar proportion of men wish to sire a child. The difference between today and the past is that, with safe, efficient contraception, the majority of couples can now choose when they will have their baby, and their parenthood can be planned.

In the general population (that is couples who have no infertility problem) the fecundity, or the capacity of a woman to become pregnant, is high: between 85 and 90 per cent of those women who wish to become pregnant will have conceived within a year, and, by 2 years, 90–95 per cent will have achieved their desired pregnancy (Fig. 1.1).

The fecundity of a woman can be defined in another way. This is a measure of her "effective" fecundity, namely the probability of a conception during a month resulting in a live birth. This has been calculated to be 30 per cent, that is, one woman in three who is fertile will become pregnant in any one month during which unprotected sexual intercourse takes place at the time of ovulation, the male also being fertile. By 4 months, 50 per cent of fertile women and, by 8 months, 70 per cent of fertile women will have become pregnant.

This means that a couple who have frequent unprotected sexual intercourse (the man ejaculating in his partner's vagina), but fail to achieve a pregnancy within 12 months of trying, should be considered to be infertile and may properly seek help if they so wish.

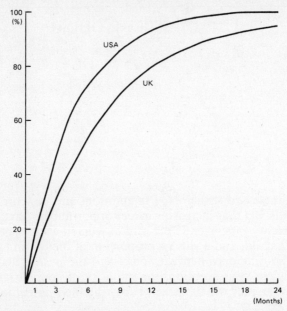

**Figure 1.1** Cumulative statistical probability of conception in a normal fertile population

It is generally estimated that between 10 and 15 per cent of couples are involuntarily childless. Although a woman's fecundity decreases after the age of 35, this is not a major cause of infertility, as most couples choose to have their baby before the woman reaches that age, and the decline, at least before the age of 40, is slight. The causes of infertility must be looked for elsewhere.

## THE ANATOMY OF INFERTILITY

Normal conception can be looked at from an anatomical viewpoint. It can be viewed by charting the journey of the sperm, until it meets the ovum; by charting the journey of the ovum; and by charting their joint journey to the uterus (Fig. 1.2).

The sperms are formed in the testicles, which are made up of long twisting tubules called seminiferous (sperm-producing) tubules (Fig. 1.3). The tubules are lined by germ cells from which the sperms develop. As they develop the cells are pushed inwards

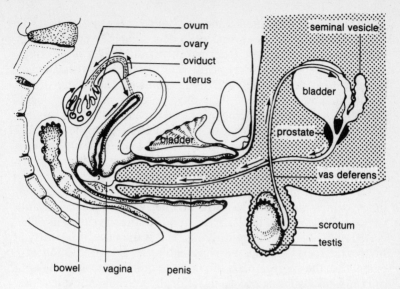

**Figure 1.2**  The journey of the sperm to reach the ovum

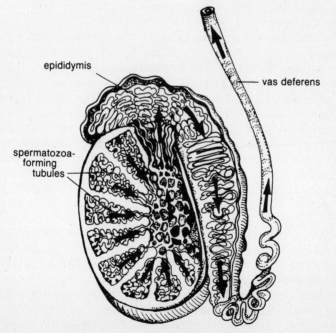

**Figure 1.3**  The testes and epididymis

into the center of the tubule and new cells are formed, so that the lining of the tubule is several cells deep. Each layer of cells is made up of spermatozoa (sperms) in various stages of development and the sperms undergo several phases of maturation or development before they are discharged into the cavity of the tubule in about 65 days. The process goes on continuously, 50 000 or more sperms being produced each minute. The tubules join together to form ducts, or tubes, along which the spermatozoa are propelled by the movement of cilia (or hairs) on the inner surface of the cells lining the ducts, because at this stage the sperms have no movement of their own.

The ducts join together to form about 12 larger collecting tubules, which then join to form a tube, which lies coiled and twisted alongside the testis, and extends to the vas deferens. The coiled tube is called the epididymis. If it is uncoiled it is nearly 6 metres (20 feet) long. If a man has regular sexual stimulation and ejaculates, the spermatozoa move quite quickly through the epididymis, taking from 7 to 10 days for the journey, but if he does not, the sperms may remain in the epididymis for much longer. The more frequently a man ejaculates, the more quickly the sperms pass along the epididymis.

The end of the epididymis joins the vas deferens, which can be identified if you put your thumb and forefinger on each side of the scrotum where it reaches the crutch, and then roll the tissues between your fingers. The vas extends from the end of the epididymis, up through the scrotum, and enters the abdomen through a weakened oval area just above the pubic bone on each side — called the inguinal canal. Inside the abdomen the vas lies close to the prostate gland, where it joins the vas from the other side. Together they enter the urethra, the tube that extends from the bladder to the eye of the penis.

Inside the epididymis, the sperms mature and are stored in the last part of the epididymis and in the vas, especially in the widened end just before it joins the urethra. The mature spermatozoa are ready to be ejaculated, mixed with secretions from two outgrowths from the widened end of the vas, called the seminal vesicles. The secretions make up the seminal fluid, which consists of millions of sperms mixed in a much larger volume of secretions from the seminal vesicles and some from the prostate gland. When ejaculated the average quantity of seminal fluid is 3 milliliters (a teaspoonful). It contains 200–500 million sperms, which accounts for about 10 per cent of its volume, the secretions making up the remaining 90 per cent.

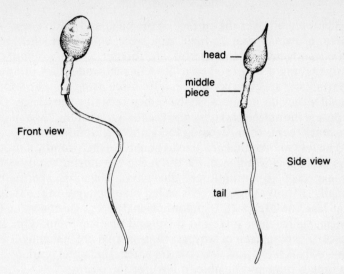

Front view

head

middle
piece

Side view

tail

**Figure 1.4**   The sperm, as seen by an electron microscope (enlarged
          × 36 000)

About 60 per cent of the secretions come from the seminal
vesicles. They contain a sugar (fructose), which gives the spermatozoa energy. Nearly all the remaining secretions come from the
prostate gland. These secretions contain various enzymes, the
concentrations of which can be measured. It has been found that
if the level of one of them, acid phosphatase, is high, and the
man's sperm count is low, he probably has a low-grade infection
of his prostate gland. This infection may be cleared up using
antibiotics, with improvement in his sperm count.

The secretions, which make up so much of the semen volume,
are important because they provide nourishment and energy for
the sperms and permit them to "exercise" their tails. Looked at
under a microscope sperms are seen to be complex (Fig. 1.4).
Each sperm has a head, a middle piece, and a tail. The head of the
sperm is shaped like the head of a snake. The head carries all the
genetic material to form a new human if it combines with genetic
material in the ovum. Covering the front of the head is a
thickened cap. Behind the head is a cylindrical midpiece, which
contains the "engine" of the sperm. The energy needed to enable
the tail of the sperm to propel it through the uterus is produced
here. The tail of the sperm is three times as long as the head and
the midpiece. The tail propels the sperm forward by a thrashing,
twisting motion.

Scattered all over the surface of the head and midpiece of the sperm are small spots, which, as it were, squirt out substances called antigens. As the sperms are foreign to the woman, the antigens might be expected to lead to the production of "antibodies" by specialized white cells circulating in her blood. Usually they do not because the semen contains substances that suppress the antigen activity and the thickness of the vaginal wall prevents them from reaching the woman's blood-stream.

The few sperms that are able to penetrate the strands of mucus that cascade down the cervix and reach the uterine cavity could be expected to "immunize" the woman against sperm, but usually do not, as special cells called macrophages in the tissues that line the uterus (the endometrium) recognize many of the sperms as foreign, surround them and destroy them. This is a possible explanation of why so many sperms are ejaculated: and why only a very few survive to reach the outer end of the Fallopian tube and be able to fertilize the ovum.

Some women appear to be especially sensitive to sperm antigens, and the protective system fails. The sperm antigens then enter the woman's tissues. When this happens she produces antibodies to sperms and is sensitized to them. When next the man ejaculates, the antibodies she is now making are ejected into the cavity of the genital tract, where they seek and cover the antigen-secreting spots on the surface of the sperms. If this happens the sperms stick together, or their tails stop thrashing so that they are immobilized and are unable to make the journey through the cervical canal and the uterus to reach the egg.

During the first part of a man's orgasm, the muscles that surround the widened ends of each of his vas deferens and his seminal vesicles contract. This forces the mixture of spermatozoa and the secretions from the prostate and the seminal vesicles along his urethra into his penis. There the muscles that surround the root of his penis start contracting and he ejaculates the seminal fluid in short spurts, and feels the pleasurable sensation of orgasm.

Once the man has deposited a sufficient quantity of healthy sperms in the woman's vagina, his contribution to conception ceases. Now the sperms have to make the voyage through the woman's genital organs to reach the egg, which by this time will be in the outer end of one of her Fallopian tubes.

A woman's vagina is a muscular tube lined by a wall of cells. The vagina stretches upwards and backwards from the external genitals to reach the uterus. Surrounding the vaginal muscles is a well-developed network of veins, which become distended in sexual arousal. Normally the walls of the vagina lie close together, the vagina being a potential cavity, which is distended by intravaginal tampons used during menstruation; by the penis at copulation; and during childbirth, when it stretches very considerably to allow the baby to be born.

The vagina is about 9 centimeters (3¾ inches) long, and at the upper end the cervix (or neck) of the uterus projects into it (Fig. 1.5). The vagina lies between the bladder in front and the rectum (or back-passage) behind. At the sides it is surrounded and protected by the strong muscles of the floor of the pelvis. Unless the vagina has been damaged, injured or tightened at operation, or has not developed due to an absence of sex hormones, its size is always adequate for sexual intercourse. A woman who menstruates has a normal-sized vagina, and difficulty at intercourse is not due to her being made small. The cause lies not in the vagina, but in a fear of sexual intercourse, which leads the woman

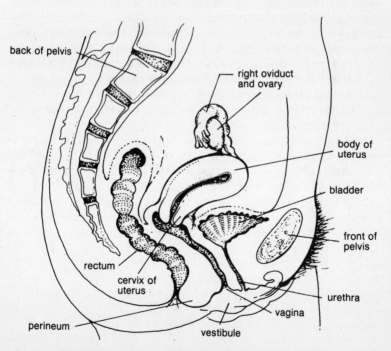

**Figure 1.5** The internal genital organs of the female

to tighten the muscles that support the vagina to such an extent that intercourse is painful. Very occasionally this prevents intercourse and is a cause of infertility.

The uterus is a hollow muscular organ lying in the middle of the woman's pelvis between the bladder in front and the bowel behind.

It is pear shaped, and averages 9 centimeters (3¾ inches) in length, 6 centimeters (2½ inches) in width at its widest part and it weighs about 60 grams (2 oz.). Viewed from in front its cavity is triangular, and it is lined with a special tissue, called the endometrium, which is made up of glands (which open onto its surface) in a meshwork of cells. For descriptive purposes, the uterus can be divided into a lower portion, the cervix (or neck), and an upper portion, called the corpus (or body) (Fig. 1.6). In the cervix the cavity is narrow, forming a canal, which is lined by cells that dip into the underlying tissue. The cells secrete mucus, which forms a thick, almost unpenetrable mesh, except at the time of ovulation when, under the influence of the female sex hormone, estrogen, the mucus is rearranged into long strands, with spiral passages between the strands. The spiral passages lead into the cavity of the body of the uterus. Normally, the uterus lies, bent forward at an angle of 90° to the vagina, resting on the bladder. As the bladder fills the uterus rotates backwards, and in 10 per cent of women it lies bent backwards, or retroverted. In the past a retroverted uterus was believed to cause infertility, but it is now known that this is not so and the operations recommended for "cure of retroversion" are rarely needed.

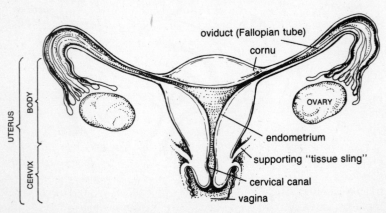

**Figure 1.6**  The cavity of the uterus, and tubes

At the upper and outer end of the pear-shaped uterus, the oviducts (or Fallopian tubes) stretch out into the pelvis. They are two small, hollow tubes, one on each side, which stretch for about 10 centimeters (4 inches) from the upper part of the uterus, to lie in contact with the ovary on each side. The outer or "fimbrial" end of each oviduct is divided into long finger-like processes, and it is thought that these sweep up the egg (or ovum) when it is expelled from the ovary. The oviduct is lined with cells shaped like goblets, which lie between cells with frond-like borders. The oviduct is of great importance, as it is within it that fertilization of the ovum takes place, and it is likely that its secretions help to nourish the fertilized ovum as it is moved by the cells with long fronds towards the uterus.

The two ovaries are ovoid-shaped organs, averaging 3½ centimeters (1½ inches) in length and 2 centimeters (¾ inch) in breadth. In the infant they are small, delicate, thin structures, but after puberty they enlarge to reach the adult proportions mentioned. After the menopause they become small and wrinkled, and in old age are less than half their adult size. Each ovary has a center made up of small cells and a mesh of vessels. Surrounding this is the ovary proper — the cortex — which contains about 200 000 egg cells lying in a cellular bed (the stroma), and outside again, protecting the egg cells and the ovarian stroma, is a thickened layer of tissue. The ovaries are the equivalent of the male testes, and in addition to containing the egg cells produce the female sex hormones, estrogen and progesterone.

As can be appreciated, the passage within the genital tract extends from the woman's vulva, along the vagina, through the cervix and uterus, and along the tubes to the ovaries. Ejaculated into the upper vagina the sperms have to journey to the outer end of the oviducts to meet the ovum.

## HOW CONCEPTION OCCURS

From the above description it can be inferred that several events have to take place for conception to occur. The most important event is that the sperm, having completed its journey, penetrates the shell of the ovum (which has completed its journey from the ovary) and fertilizes it. Two or three days later, the fertilized egg moves down the oviduct to reach the uterus, where it may implant. Not all fertilized eggs implant. In normal fertile couples, who do not use contraceptives, it has been calculated that 30 per cent of fertilized ova fail to implant into the endometrium. This information is important when judging the efficacy of *in-vitro* fertilization and embryo transplantation. In simple terms the required conditions and the sequence of events that lead to a pregnancy are as follows:

- The woman must be able to ovulate. The ovum that has developed in one of the follicles in her ovary must have been released and been taken up by the finger-like processes at the outer end of her oviduct. Obviously if she fails to ovulate or if the ovum is not able to enter the oviduct, pregnancy will not occur.
- The man must be able to produce a reasonable quantity of healthy spermatozoa in his semen.
- The man has to be able to obtain and maintain an erection of his penis and to ejaculate the semen, containing the healthy sperms, into the upper part of the woman's vagina.
- Unprotected sexual intercourse should take place sufficiently frequently for ejaculation to occur about the time the woman ovulates.
- Some of the ejaculated sperms (which number several hundred million) have to swim through the spiral channels in the mucus of the woman's cervix to enter her uterus.
- The sperms, now reduced in numbers, have to swim through the uterus and enter the tunnel of the woman's oviducts. Obviously if the environment in the uterus is abnormal, or if the oviducts are damaged or blocked, the journey of the sperms will be halted.
- A sperm has to come into contact with the ovum in the oviduct within 12 hours of ovulation and its head (which carries the genetic material) must enter the substance of the ovum to fertilize it.
- The fertilized egg has then to pass along the oviduct to enter the cavity of the uterus, and has to implant onto its inner lining (or endometrium).

## INVESTIGATING INFERTILITY

The investigation of an infertile couple is to determine which of the events just outlined is not occurring. You will note that it is the *couple* who are investigated. Preferably they should be investigated simultaneously, but usually the woman first presents because she has failed to become pregnant.

Many complex series of investigations have been suggested but are often counter-productive as they increase the anxiety of the couple, and this, in turn, may hinder conception. In reality a fairly simple approach, requiring two or three visits, is sufficient to establish what the problem is.

At the first visit the woman is asked about her general health, previous illnesses or operations, and whether she has ever been pregnant. If she has never been pregnant she is said to have *primary infertility*, whereas if she has previously been pregnant she has *secondary infertility*.

She is asked about her menstrual history, particularly when menstruation started, the frequency of her menstrual periods, whether or not she has menstrual cramps (dysmenorrhoea), and whether or not she has a vaginal discharge.

She is asked about her sexual activity, particular attention being placed on the frequency of sexual intercourse, whether she feels her husband or partner ejaculate within her vagina, and her attitudes to her sexuality.

After taking a medical history and a sexual history, the doctor examines the woman physically. If she has had a general physical check in the previous months the doctor may omit this, but will need to examine her abdomen and do a pelvic examination.

At the end of these examinations (which usually reveal no abnormalities) the doctor invites the woman to bring her husband or partner so that the sequence of the proposed investigations may be outlined. Although there is no *medical* need for the man to attend at this stage, provided sexual intercourse is regular and satisfactory and provided he is willing to provide a sample of his semen for analysis, there are psychological advantages for the couple to be seen together.

At the initial visit, the doctor may invite the woman to take her temperature each morning before rising and to chart it for 1 or 2 months. This is one of the ways to determine if she is ovulating, which is discussed in detail in Chapter 2. Although, as will be seen, it is not a very accurate method, it has the advantage of involving the couple in their own treatment. At the same visit, the doctor invites the woman to ask her husband or partner to provide a specimen of his semen for analysis, as is discussed in Chapter 3. Some doctors also invite her to attend at the probable time of ovulation, having had intercourse about 6 hours earlier, for a postcoital test. This is discussed in Chapter 4. Other doctors doubt the value of this test.

When it has been established that the man has normal semen and that intravaginal ejaculation takes place, it is usual to arrange for the next step in the investigations. This is to determine whether the woman's uterus and oviducts are normal in shape and whether or not there is a block, which may prevent the sperm from reaching the ovum. Two tests are available to find out the answer to these questions. The first is a simple procedure, the second more complex and invasive. For the first procedure the woman is asked to attend an X ray department. There the doctor introduces a speculum into her vagina, so that he can see her cervix. He inserts a narrow tube into the cervix. This is connected to a syringe containing a watery or oily dye that is opaque to X rays. The woman lies under an X ray machine and the picture of her pelvic organs is relayed to a television screen so that she and the doctor can see what happens when he injects the dye. Usually it fills the uterus and then passes along the oviducts and drips into her pelvis. The procedure is not painful and takes about 5 minutes. It is called a hysterosalpingogram.

The second procedure is to admit the woman to hospital for a day and to inspect her pelvic organs by making a tiny cut just below her umbilicus, and inserting a telescope-like instrument called a laparoscope. This is done under a general anesthetic, and the woman usually experiences some discomfort for a few hours (or longer) when she wakes up from the anesthetic.

Although some doctors omit doing a hysterosalpingogram and only do a laparoscopy, most would agree that a hysterosalpingogram should be done first, and the laparoscope reserved for women whose hysterosalpingogram is abnormal. These matters are considered in Chapter 7.

This investigation completes the basic investigations for infertility, and other, more complex, investigations are only required in special circumstances.

The investigations outlined will establish a reason for the couple's inability to conceive a child in about 75–85 per cent of cases. In the remaining cases, no reason can be found and the infertility is unexplained. This is considered in Chapter 10.

## CAUSES OF INFERTILITY

In a given population the relative proportions of the causes of infertility will vary, depending on the country and social class of the couples. For example, in some southern European and Asian countries, tuberculosis of the uterus and oviducts is the cause of infertility in about 5 per cent of women, whereas in Australia, genital tuberculosis is rarely seen. In Central Africa, chronic infection of the Fallopian tubes, caused by gonorrhoea, is a significant cause of infertility, but in Western nations, gonorrhoea is an infrequent cause, although pelvic infection due to other germs occurs. Another variable is that in about 10 per cent of couples presenting with infertility, multiple causes are present. For example, the man may have a low sperm count and the woman may only ovulate infrequently. Despite these variables a consensus can be obtained enabling the relative frequency of the causes of infertility to be classified, and an estimate to be given of the chance of pregnancy occurring following investigations and treatment (Table 1.1). It is surprising, and currently inexplicable,

**Table 1.1  Factors involved in infertility\***

| Infertility problem | Proportion[†] of total number (%) (Range) | Pregnancy rate (with or without treatment) (%) |
|---|---|---|
| Disordered ovulation | 21 (10–40) | 60–90 |
| Male factors (mainly sperm defects) | 32 (10–35) | 35–75 Using AID as treatment |
| Cervical and immunological | 5 (3–8) | 10–20 |
| Tubal and uterine | 19 (10–30) | 15–50 |
| Unexplained | 23 (5–40) | 30–60 With or without treatment |

\*If several factors are involved, the main one is recorded.
†Proportional percentage and range derived from 10 reports of series of 400 or more couples investigated.

that in several studies between 15 and 25 per cent of women who have been infertile for 2 or more years become pregnant either during or within 4 months of completion of the investigations and before any treatment has been given. Some doctors argue that investigation is treatment, giving as an example the suggestion that the injection of the dye under pressure during a hysterosalpingogram may break fine adhesions that obstruct the oviduct. Other doctors note that some anovulatory women begin ovulating before they are given fertility drugs. In a study in Melbourne, Australia, of 545 women who were not ovulating, over half ovulated and one-third became pregnant when given placebo (sugar) pills before fertility pills were prescribed. In IVF programs, when there is a delay of weeks or months between entering the program and the first IVF attempt, about 5 per cent of women become pregnant before the first IVF attempt if the woman was put on the program for reasons other than damaged Fallopian tubes.

It is clear from these findings that the understanding of infertility is still incomplete and much rigorous research is needed.

What the couple want to know is the answer to the question: "What are our chances of having a live, healthy baby?" A study of Tables 1.1 and 1.2 shows that the pregnancy rate (and the "take home baby" rate) depends on the main infertility problem identified. But, overall, if 100 infertile couples are investigated and offered appropriate treatment, 40–50 per cent may expect to be pregnant within 2 years. This is considered at greater length in Chapter 12.

**Table 1.2   Outcome of investigation and treatment for infertility***

| Infertility factor | Percentage of total number | Pregnancy rate (%) | Pregnancy per 100 couples |
|---|---|---|---|
| Male factors | 32 | 40 | 13 |
| Ovulation disorders | 21 | 57 | 12 |
| Tubal (and uterine) | 19 | 24 | 4.5 |
| Cervical/immunological | 5 | 14 | 0.7 |
| Unexplained | 23 | 60 | 13.8 |
| | | | 44.0 |

*Based on several series totalling over 3000 couples.

# 2

# Disorders of Ovulation

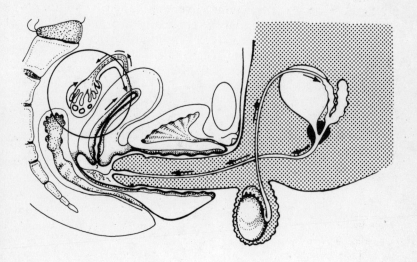

# 2

# Disorders of Ovulation

Ovulation occurs in most but not all menstrual cycles of most women who are aged between 17 and 40. At the extremes of the reproductive years (i.e. under the age of 17 and over the age of 40) ovulation is less frequent. In about 20 per cent of infertile women, ovulation fails to occur, or if it does occur, the normal hormone levels consequent upon ovulation do not eventuate, with the result that the ovum, even if fertilized, is unable to implant on an improperly prepared endometrium. The soil is too poor! These conditions constitute the disorders of ovulation, and they may be accompanied clinically by amenorrhea, which can be defined as menstruation occurring at intervals of more than 6 months, or by infrequent periods (oligomenorrhea), which is defined as menstrual intervals greater than 6 weeks but less than 6 months. In a few women with ovulatory disturbances, the menstrual periods are regular but ovulation fails to occur regularly or does not occur at all. This is termed anovulation.

The release of an ovum from the ovary (ovulation) occurring at regular intervals depends on an interplay between hormones released from the lower part of the brain (the hypothalamus), the pituitary gland and ovary itself (Fig. 2.1). The hypothalamus synthesizes and releases a hormone called the gonadotrophin-releasing hormone, or GnRH. Under the influence of GnRH the pituitary gland secretes and releases two hormones that act on the gonads (ovaries). These are follicle-stimulating hormone (FSH) and luteinizing hormone (LH). They are called gonadotrophic hormones because they induce the gonads to grow and produce hormones. The ovaries in turn produce the female sex hormones, estrogen and progesterone.

23

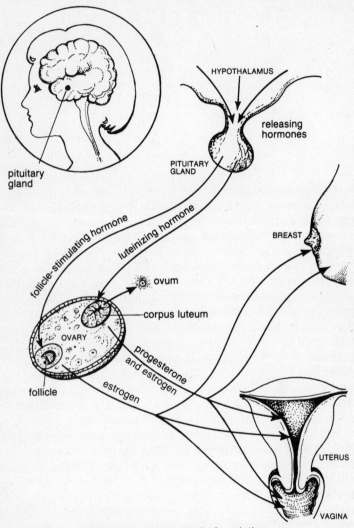

**Figure 2.1**  The control of ovulation

   The sequence of events leading to ovulation is complicated, and can best be understood if the description starts at the onset of menstruation as this is a significant event, each month, in most women's lives. During menstruation the hypothalamus sends quantities of GnRH, in pulsatile surges, to stimulate the cells in the pituitary gland that manufacture FSH. The amount of FSH in the blood rises and stimulates a number of egg follicles in the ovary, usually 12–20. As these follicles grow they synthesize estrogen, so that the quantity of this female sex hormone increases in the blood. Estrogen has several effects on the tissues that make up the genital tract, one of which being its action on the lining (endometrium) of the uterus. Estrogen stimulates the endometrium to grow. At the end of menstruation most of the endometrium has crumbled away and, mixed with blood and tissue fluid, has been shed as the menstrual flow. The endometrium is made up of narrow tubes, called endometrial glands, set in several layers of supporting cells, called endometrial stromal cells. Estrogen stimulates the growth and development of endometrial glands and the supporting stromal cells, which increase in numbers (proliferate). This is why this part of the menstrual cycle is called the proliferative phase of the cycle.

As the level of estrogen rises in the blood, it "feeds back" to the hypothalamus to reduce the amount of FSH released, so that the system is kept under control. Then, about 2 weeks after the start of the menstrual period, estrogen is released from the follicles in a sudden surge. This raises its level in the blood four-fold for a few hours. This high level of estrogen feeds back to the hypothalamus in a unique way, inducing it to release a second gonadotrophic hormone called luteinizing hormone releasing hormone (LHRH). LHRH is carried to the pituitary gland in blood vessels that connect the two parts of the brain, where it induces the sudden production of luteinizing hormone (LH). A surge of LH is released into the blood and is carried to the ovaries, where it acts on the largest egg follicle, which by now has moved through the ovary to reach its surface, where it makes a tiny bulge that can be seen by the naked eye. Under the influence of the luteinizing hormone, the follicle bursts and the ovum is pushed out, together with the fluid in which it lay. The ovum is caught in the fingerlike ends of the oviduct, which caress the ovary at this time, and is moved slowly but gently into the cavity of the Fallopian tube, where fertilization takes place, if this is to happen (Fig. 2.2).

Once the ovum has been expelled, the now empty follicle collapses, and the luteinizing hormone acts on the cells of its wall, turning them yellow. The collapsed follicle is called a yellow body, or, in Latin, a *corpus luteum*. The change in color of the cells of the corpus luteum is due to a change in their activity. Now, not only do they continue to secrete estrogen (together with the cells of the other 11–19 stimulated follicles, which failed to

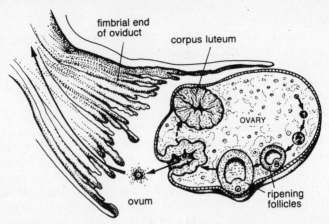

**Figure 2.2** Growth of stimulated follicles in the ovary during a menstrual cycle

grow so quickly), but uniquely they also manufacture a hormone called progesterone. The name is apt, for the hormone prepares the uterus for pregnancy (*progestos*), hence pro-gest-erone (-*one* indicates the kind of chemical substance). Progesterone is the second main female sex hormone. It has many actions, but the main ones are that it relaxes smooth (involuntary) muscles, increases the production of the waxy secretions of the skin and raises the temperature of the body. This is why it is normal for women in the second half of the menstrual cycle to have a temperature up to 37.4°C (99.5°F). The most important progestational effect of progesterone is its action on the uterus. Progesterone thickens the lining of the uterus, and induces the glands to secrete a nutritious fluid and become succulent, so that the fertilized egg may be nourished during the time it needs to implant in the lining of the uterus. The part of the menstrual cycle after ovulation is called the luteal or the progestational phase (Fig. 2.3).

Unless the egg is fertilized and implants into the endometrium, the yellow body in the ovary dies (as do the other stimulated follicles). When this happens, the levels of estrogen and progesterone in the blood fall. This has two effects: first, the restraint on GnRH production by the hypothalamus is removed, and FSH production by the pituitary gland increases. Secondly, without the stimulation of estrogen and progesterone, the now thick, juicy lining of the uterus begins to shrink, and in doing so kinks

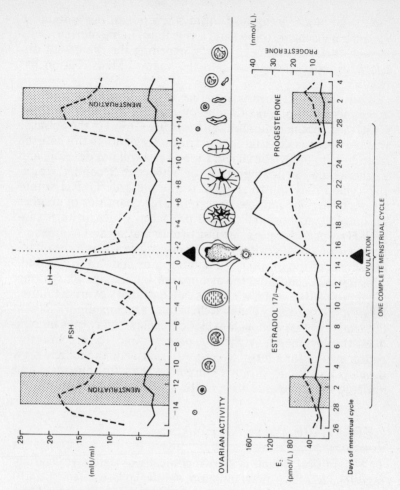

**Figure 2.3** The hormonal relationships of the menstrual cycle (from Derek Llewellyn-Jones: Fundamentals of Obstetrics and Gynaecology Vol 1, 5th Edition, 1990 London: Faber & Faber by permission)

the tiny blood capillary vessels, which release substances called prostaglandins. These in turn make the blood capillaries contract and then dilate. This causes them to break, and patchy bleeding occurs in the deeper layers of the endometrium, which crumbles and is shed into the uterine cavity, together with blood and tissue fluid. The blood clots, but quickly the clots are dissolved so that menstrual blood is liquid. Within a few hours, the amount of menstrual discharge (blood and tissue fluid) in the uterine cavity is such that the uterus contracts, expelling the menstrual discharge through the cervix into the vagina. Menstruation has begun.

Because of the reciprocal nature of the hormonal feedback mechanisms, disorders of ovulation may occur at several levels. First, the hypothalamus may fail to release GnRH in the pulsatile manner necessary to stimulate the pituitary gland. In this case the ovaries will not be stimulated, the follicles will not develop, and neither ovulation nor menstruation will occur. Second, the pituitary gland may fail to respond to the pulsatile GnRH stimulation; or may be induced to secrete large quantities of another pituitary gland hormone, called prolactin, which in turn suppresses ovarian function, leading to anovulation and to amenorrhea. Third, the ovary itself may be insensitive to, or resistant to, the effects of the pituitary gonadotrophins and fail to respond. This is what occurs after the menopause, but it may occur during the reproductive years, when it is called primary ovarian failure. Fourth, the most stimulated follicle may develop abnormally in the ovary, so that although ovulation occurs, the corpus luteum does not synthesize sufficient progesterone to prepare the endometrium for a fertilized egg. Alternatively, the follicle may develop but fail to rupture, trapping the ovum, but may still undergo the changes leading to the synthesis of progesterone.

## DEFECTIVE LUTEAL PHASE

This condition, which is known clinically as defective ovarian function, defective luteal function, or luteal phase defect, is diagnosed with varying frequency by different investigators. The precise diagnosis is difficult because it depends on knowing accurately, first, when ovulation has occurred so that the beginning of the luteal phase can be identified precisely and, second, obtaining evidence that the luteal phase is defective. Many investigators have made the assumption that ovulation always occurs 12 – 15 days before the first day of the next menstrual period, and that a luteal phase that is shorter than 11 days indicates defective luteal function. Although this "fact" has been accepted for at least 20 years, it now appears that ovulation may occur between 17 and 10 days before the onset of menstruation in fertile women.

This makes suspect the assumption that a short luteal phase is defective.

To find out whether the luteal phase is defective, other methods must be used. Two ways of determining this have been suggested. The first is for the doctor to take a sample of the endometrium by introducing a small instrument through the cervix. The sample is examined by a pathologist who uses certain changes in the tissues to date it and to decide if a lag of more than 2 days in its expected development is present. There are problems about this as the appearance of the endometrium is subjective, and different pathologists date the same piece of endometrium differently. For this reason many authorities would only accept that the luteal phase is defective if the lag were found in three menstrual cycles. Unfortunately many gynecologists fail to keep to this criterion and diagnose the condition if one sample of the endometrium is out of phase. This questions whether the defective luteal phase is a real factor in infertility, or if it is a doctor-inspired disorder.

A more accurate, but rather impractical, way of detecting possible defective luteal function is for the woman to have a blood sample taken daily for the last 2 weeks of her menstrual cycle. The levels of the hormones, estrogen and progesterone, are measured and compared with the levels found in apparently normal menstrual cycles. If an abnormal pattern is found, defective ovarian function or defective luteal phase is presumed to exist. A possible compromise is to measure the progesterone level in the mid-luteal phase, that is between 9 and 4 days before menstruation, and if the level is low (less than 21 nanomoles per liter) to take a sample of the endometrium to detect if a lag is present.

However, it should be remembered that as many pregnancies occur in untreated women who have been diagnosed as having a defective luteal phase, as among women whose luteal phase is normal.

## DIAGNOSING OVULATION

If a woman is not menstruating, for whatever reason, it is unlikely that she is ovulating. If she menstruates infrequently (or menstruates regularly but no other reason for the couple's infertility problem has been found), the decision may be made to determine if she is ovulating.

This can be done by: (1) recording the woman's basal body temperature, (2) measuring the level of progesterone in her blood 9 – 4 days before menstruation, (3) examining the ovaries using ultrasound, (4) looking at a sample of cervical mucus, or (5) taking an endometrial biopsy. The fourth and fifth tests have largely been superseded, as the fourth is not very accurate and the fifth is unpleasant for the woman.

## 1  BASAL BODY TEMPERATURE (BBT)

In this method, the woman records her temperature each morning before getting out of bed, and before having a hot drink or sex. She records the result on a sheet of graph paper. This produces a pattern, which may show that she is ovulating (Fig. 2.4). As men-

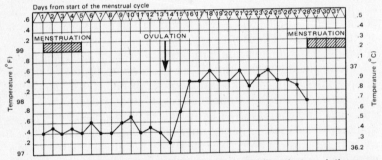

**Figure 2.4**   A biphasic temperature chart indicating that ovulation was presumed to have occurred on day 14 of the cycle

tioned earlier, progesterone leads to an increase in the basal (resting) body temperature. If the woman has ovulated, progesterone is produced by her ovaries and the chart will show a sustained rise in temperature of about 1 degree Celsius. The chart will also give an indication on which day ovulation occurred. This is at the deep point of the temperature curve, or during the rise. Unfortunately measuring the BBT has several disadvantages: in some cases the graph is difficult to interpret, some women ovulate without showing the typical ovulation pattern, a few women become fixated on their charts. These women chart their BBT for months and only have sexual intercourse on fertile days rather than when they are sexually aroused. The thermometer becomes more important than their relationship with their partner.

Inspection of BBT charts gives a reasonable indication that ovulation has occurred and when it occurred, in about 80 per cent of women using the method. However, many doctors no longer ask women to chart the BBT, preferring other methods.

## 2   SERUM PROGESTERONE LEVEL

The fact that ovulation has occurred can be diagnosed by measuring the level of progesterone in the woman's blood (or, more recently, her saliva) in the second half of her menstrual cycle. The level of progesterone rises after ovulation, and remains high until 2 or 3 days before menstruation (Fig. 2.5). This means the test can be made on any convenient day, 9–4 days before menstruation is expected. Because some women do not ovulate every menstrual cycle, serum progesterone should be measured in several cycles before the woman is informed that she is not ovulating.

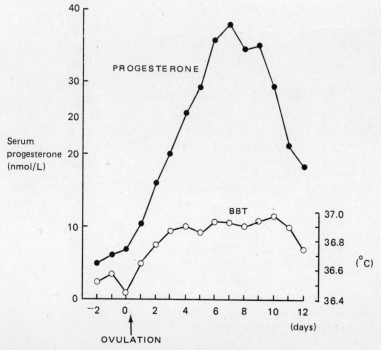

**Figure 2.5**   The rise in the level of progesterone in the blood following ovulation (BBT = basal body temperature)

## 3   ULTRASOUND

The development of sophisticated ultrasound machines has enabled the growth of the follicle to be studied. If the woman is able to attend for production of a daily ultrasound picture from about the 12th day of her cycle, the main follicle can be measured. When it measures more than 20 millimeters, ovulation is imminent. If an ultrasound picture 1 or 2 days later shows that a corpus luteum has formed, ovulation can be diagnosed.

## 4   FERNING

If a sample of the cervical mucus is taken at ovulation time, in the mid-cycle, and allowed to dry on a microscope slide, a "fern" pattern will appear in women who have ovulated (Fig. 2.6). Two days after ovulation the fern pattern disappears as progesterone alters the character of the cervical mucus.

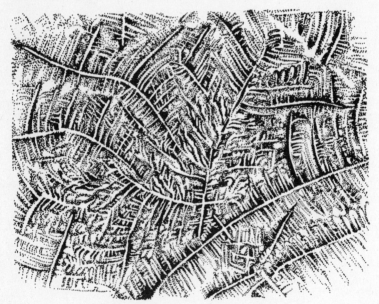

**Figure 2.6**   Cervical mucus ferning

## 5   ENDOMETRIAL BIOPSY

Until accurate hormone assays for progesterone in the blood became available, doctors often took a sample of the endometrium (usually about 2 days before the expected day of menstruation) by inserting a narrow curette into the woman's uterus and scraping off a sliver of endometrium from the upper part of the uterine cavity. The procedure was uncomfortable, but women were prepared to put up with it. The specimen was sent to a laboratory, and looked at through a microscope.

The appearance of the endometrial glands and the supporting tissues, or stroma, alter under the influence of estrogen and progesterone. The glands become twisted and secrete fluid into the cavity of the uterus. The altered appearance enables a pathologist to infer that ovulation has occurred.

# INVESTIGATING DISORDERS OF OVULATION

The absence of ovulation (anovulation) or the failure of the corpus luteum to function properly (called ovulation defect, defective luteal function, or luteal insufficiency) is a cause of infertility in between 10 and 20 per cent of couples who present to a doctor. About half of the women will have amenorrhea, that is an absence of menstruation for 6 months or longer; more than one-third will have menstrual periods at intervals of 6 weeks to 6 months (oligomenorrhea), most or all of which are anovulatory; and a few women will be found to have defective ovarian function (defective luteal function), if this is a real condition.

The investigation of infertile women who have disorders of ovulation is made in several stages, so that a particular disorder may be indentified and treatment offered.

## 1  HISTORY

The doctor takes a history of the woman's menstrual pattern from puberty onwards and scrutinizes it, to see if any pointers emerge. Her weight is noted and she is questioned about her eating habits. It is known that women who are considerably underweight due to dieting or to anorexia nervosa and women who are bulimic, alternating binge-eating with behaviors to induce weight loss (such as self-induced vomiting, laxative or diuretic abuse and starvation dieting) usually cease to ovulate, as do some obese women. The woman's exercise habits are discussed, as women who exercise excessively also tend to cease to ovulate. The doctor enquires about contraceptive methods used by the woman, since a few women (between 4 and 7 per 1000) who have stopped taking the pill for a year or more continue to fail to ovulate and usually also fail to menstruate.

## 2  CLINICAL EXAMINATION

The woman is examined clinically to check her general health, and the condition of her genital organs. The doctor notes if she is overweight and examines her for excess hair (hirsutism) as some women who have oligomenorrhea (occasionally amenorrhea) and who are overweight and hirsute, have a condition called "the polycystic ovarian syndrome," which may be a cause of infertility. However, not all women who have polycystic ovaries are overweight or hirsute.

## 3  ULTRASOUND AND X RAYS

Ultrasound, particularly if a vaginal probe is used, enables doctors to scan the ovaries and to detect polycystic ovaries with greater accuracy. Most doctors also recommend that an X ray of the pituitary area of the skull is taken in women who have had amenorrhea for 6 months or more. This is to make sure that a pituitary tumor is not the cause of amenorrhea.

## 4  HORMONE TESTS

Many tests, some simple, some very complicated, have been devised to investigate women who have disorders of ovulation. Most of these tests are only needed for research and a relatively simple group of tests will provide the information needed to be able to treat nearly all the disorders of ovulation associated with infertility. If a woman has amenorrhea or oligomenorrhea, a small amount of blood is taken and the level of three hormones is measured. The hormones are the follicle-stimulating hormone (FSH), the prolactin hormone (PRL) and the thyroid-stimulating hormone (TSH). If the woman is thought to have polycystic ovarian disease, the level of luteinizing hormone (LH) is also measured (Fig. 2.7).

The woman is given tablets of a synthetic progesterone, medroxy progesterone acetate (MPA). She is asked to take one tablet twice a day for 5 days. The purpose of this test, called the "progesterone challenge test," is to determine dynamically whether the woman has a certain amount of estrogen circulating in her blood and whether her uterus will respond to the sex hormones.

X-ray skull and measure blood hormones:

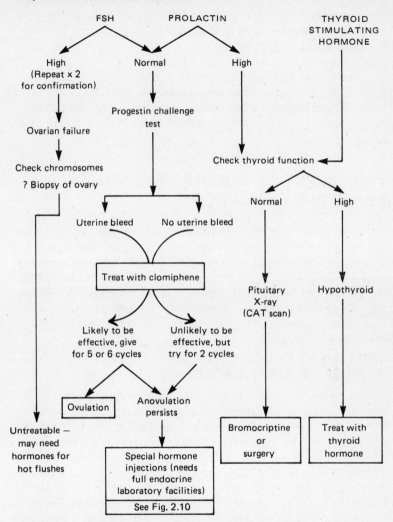

**Figure 2.7** Principles of treatment of amenorrhea, oligomenorrhea: woman's weight in normal range, no evidence of polycystic ovaries

The test depends on the fact that unless the endometrium has been stimulated to grow by estrogen, progesterone given for a few days and then stopped will not lead to uterine bleeding. If uterine

bleeding occurs in 4 days after the MPA dosage stops, the progesterone challenge test is positive and it is likely that a relatively
simple drug regimen will induce ovulation. If uterine bleeding
does not occur, it is probable that a complicated drug regimen
will be needed to induce ovulation.

If the woman has oligomenorrhea and the hormone levels are
normal or if she is menstruating regularly, blood is taken between
9 and 4 days before her expected menstruation and the level of
progesterone in the sample is measured to find out if she is ovulating.

# TREATMENT OF ANOVULATION AND DEFECTIVE OVULATION

After the doctor has evaluated the woman's history and has had
the results of the hormone tests, the reason for her failure to
ovulate should be apparent. The doctor should explain the results
to the couple and discuss the appropriate treatment to induce
ovulation. The principles of the treatment are shown in Figures
2.8 to 2.11, and the following may help the couple to understand
what is proposed.

## TREATMENT OF HYPOTHALAMIC MALFUNCTION AS A CAUSE OF ANOVULATION

In about 50 per cent of women with ovulatory disorders the problem lies in the hypothalamus, which fails to release the pulsatile
surges of GnRH needed to stimulate the pituitary gland to release
FSH and LH. The common reasons for the failure are eating disorders (anorexia nervosa, bulimia or binge-eating, and obesity);
excessive exercise (Fig. 2.8); the use of the "pill" or for a period
after taking oral contraceptives; some drugs (especially tranquil-
lizers); and psychological problems, such as depression. Women
who have anorexia nervosa, bulimia, or who are obese and anovulatory usually begin to ovulate once they change their eating
behavior and gain weight (or reduce weight, if obesity is the
problem) so that their weight falls within the desirable range. No
other treatment is required, and if offered, may cause problems if
the woman becomes pregnant. Similarly, women who exercise
excessively will resume ovulating when they reduce the amount
of exercise.

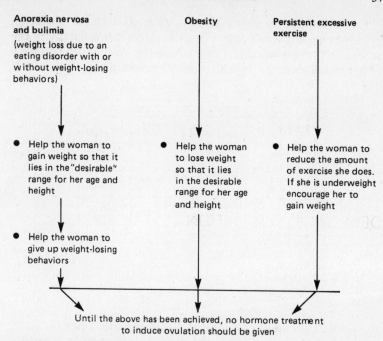

**Figure 2.8**   Principles of treatment of amenorrhea or oligomenorrhea: women who have an eating disorder or are compulsive exercisers

## Clomiphene

Women whose weight is normal and who exercise normally usually begin to ovulate if treated with the fertility drug, clomiphene. However, it is appropriate to wait for a few months after the investigations are completed, before giving clomiphene, as between 10 and 30 per cent of the women will ovulate or become pregnant during this time, without any treatment. Clomiphene tablets are taken by mouth for 5 days each month. As different women respond differently to clomiphene, it is usual for the doctor to prescribe a small dose initially (50 milligrams each day) and to increase the dose each month to a maximum of 250 milligrams a day if ovulation does not occur. The purpose of the initial small dose and gradual increase is to avoid multiple ovulation and multiple pregnancy as far as possible, although twins occur in about 10 per cent of women who require clomiphene to induce ovulation.

Ovulation occurs about 10 days after starting the course of clomiphene, if it is to occur. For this reason it is usual to ask the woman to have a blood test to measure the level of progesterone in her blood about 21 days after starting clomiphene (Fig. 2.9). If

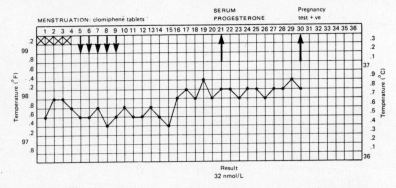

**Figure 2.9**   Basal body temperature recovery after treatment with clomiphene indicating that ovulation has occurred

the level of progesterone indicates that ovulation has occurred and pregnancy fails to occur, the same dose is given for a further month; but if ovulation has not occurred, the dose of clomiphene is increased the next month. If after 4–6 months of treatment with increasing doses of clomiphene, ovulation has not occurred, other fertility drugs may be suggested, after an interval of 3–6 months without treatment. This interval is recommended as spontaneous ovulation and pregnancy occur in some women following the use of clomiphene.

Clomiphene acts on the hypothalamus, causing it to release GnRH in pulsatile surges, which initiates the sequence of hormonal events leading to ovulation. Occasionally the sequence leads to the development of a large follicle, which fails to release its contained ovum, and an injection of a gonadotrophin containing LH is required. The drug is obtained from the urine of pregnant women, and is called human chorionic gonadotrophin (HCG).

## Hormone treatment

If clomiphene (with or without HCG) fails to induce ovulation the woman needs to be referred to a special clinic that has an endocrine laboratory.

1  Give injections of human menopausal gonadotrophin (HMG), monitoring the development of the follicle by measuring the level of estradiol in blood, estrogens in urine or by daily ultrasound examinations of the ovary. When ovulation is estimated to be about to occur, an injection of human chorionic gonadotrophin (HCG) is given to induce ovulation

↓

If the above treatment fails to induce ovulation after 3 attempts

↓

2  Give subcutaneous or intravenous injections of gonadotrophic releasing hormone (GnRH) by a portable battery-driven pump. This delivers regulated doses of GnRH every 90 minutes for 15–20 days

**Figure 2.10**  Principles of treatment when anovulation persists despite use of clomiphene

Three approaches have been developed. These are (1) injections of human menopausal gonadotrophin (HMG) and human chorionic gonadotrophin (HCG), (2) periodic injections of gonadotrophin-releasing hormone (GnRH), (3) injections of human pituitary gonadotrophin (HPG) and HCG.

**Gonadotrophin-releasing hormone**  This is the most recently developed treatment and will probably replace the other two treatments as more experience is gained. The advantage of GnRH treatment is that the hormone induces the gonadotrophin cells in the pituitary gland to release appropriate amounts of FSH and LH, and the amount released is controlled by a "built-in feed-back." This means that overstimulation of the ovaries and multiple ovulations are largely avoided, and the daily monitoring of estrogen levels required by the other two methods is not necessary.

The hormone is injected into the subcutaneous tissues of the upper abdomen or into a vein in the forearm, every 90 minutes for a period of 15–20 days by an automatic portable pump. This method enables the woman to live a relatively normal life during treatment. The dose seems critical and may depend on the degree of hypothalamic failure. This can be determined, to some extent, by measuring the levels of FSH and LH in the woman's blood before starting treatment.

Ovulation is detected by ultrasound examinations, and following ovulation, the injections of GnRH are continued for a further 12 days or so, to make sure that the endometrium develops properly and is receptive to the fertilized egg.

After treatment with GnRH, sometimes for 2 or 3 months, about 80 per cent of patients achieve a pregnancy.

**HMG and HCG treatment** Human menopausal gonadotrophin, HMG (Humegon, Pergonal), is produced from the urine of menopausal women. HMG consists mostly of FSH with additional LH, usually in the form of human chorionic gonadotrophin (HCG) obtained from the urine of pregnant women. This is added to standardize the drug so that the ratio of FSH to LH is one to one. This has been found to be the most effective ratio to obtain growth of some of the follicles.

The HMG stimulates the growth of egg follicles, but each egg will not be released from its follicle, in other words ovulation will not occur, until the swollen follicle has been stimulated to burst by an injection of HCG which produces a sudden rise in the second gonadotrophic hormone, luteinizing hormone, LH. (See p. 25).

HMG is injected each day for about 7 days and the level of estrogen in the blood is measured daily. The level of estrogen determines the amount of HMG needed the following day. When the level of estrogen in the blood or the urine rises to lie in the range expected to occur prior to ovulation and ultrasound shows the ovaries to contain no more than two large follicles, a "boosting" injection of HCG is given to induce ovulation 36–40 hours later. However, if the level of estrogen lies outside the normal range the booster injection is withheld. After an interval of a week or so, a further series of injections are started.

It will be obvious that the cost of the drugs, the cost of the laboratory investigations, and the costs of the medical care mean that HMG and HCG should only be prescribed by "super-specialists."

**HPG and HCG treatment** Before GnRH treatment became available, some women who failed to ovulate following clomiphene and then HMG + HCG treatment were offered treatment with human pituitary gonadotrophin (HPG) obtained from pituitary glands of people who had died following injury or accidents. HPG is extremely expensive to produce and is in short supply. The treatment regimen is similar to that of HMG, but with HPG replacing HMG. Like the HMG + HCG treatment, HPG + HCG treatment will probably be replaced by GnRH treatment, except for a very small number of women whose pituitary gland has been damaged, so that it cannot respond to GnRH. About 70 per cent of women become pregnant following treatment with HMG + HCG or HPG + HCG.

## TREATMENT OF HYPERPROLACTINEMIA AS A CAUSE OF ANOVULATION

In about 30 per cent of women the investigations will show that the cause of the anovulation (and usually amenorrhea) is a high level of circulating prolactin (hyperprolactinemia). Many of these women also secrete milk if their breasts are stimulated. The hyperprolactinemia is due to an overgrowth of the cells in the pituitary gland that synthesize and secrete prolactin. The cells may form a tumor, and this is investigated by radiology of the pituitary area of the brain (usually by a CAT scan) before prescribing treatment. Smaller tumors (and most larger tumors) are treated by drugs that prevent the cells secreting prolactin. The commonly used drug is called bromocriptine, which is taken by mouth in tablet form. The cells shrink in size, the level of prolactin in the blood falls and ovulation occurs.

Bromocriptine is taken with meals twice a day and is started in a small dose (1.25 milligrams) to avoid gastric upsets and to help the woman become accustomed to the drug. The amount is doubled after a week. Three weeks after treatment was started the blood levels of prolactin, estrogen and progesterone are measured to determine if a response has occurred. The level of prolactin is expected to fall, that of estrogen to rise, and if ovulation occurs, the level of progesterone will rise. If there is no response, as judged by the hormone levels, the dose of bromocriptine is doubled to 5 milligrams twice a day and the response is again tested about 3 weeks later. Most women respond by ovulating at a daily dose of 5 or 10 milligrams and most become pregnant within 6 months.

## TREATMENT OF POLYCYSTIC OVARIAN SYNDROME AS A CAUSE OF ANOVULATION

Between 5 and 10 per cent of women with ovulation disorders and infertility will be found to have the polycystic ovarian syndrome (Figure 2.11). Although hormone treatment will usually induce ovulation, it will not alter the woman's hairiness or her obesity.

Treatment of the polycystic ovarian syndrome remains controversial. Most specialists give either clomiphene or the HMG + HCG treatment described on p. 40. These treatments lead to ovulation in over 60 per cent of women, but fewer than 20 per cent become pregnant. This is thought to be because the woman's own sex hormones, which are disturbed in the disorder, interfere with the action of the prescribed hormones, so that the uterus is not properly prepared for the fertilized egg. To counter the effect of the woman's hormones some specialists suppress her sex hormone secretion by asking the woman to sniff a gonado-trophin analogue (see p. 156) 5 times daily, or to have a daily injection of it for a number of days. This effectively suppresses the secretion of her own sex hormones. When this has occurred the woman is given HMG + HCG. Reports show that 50 per cent of women with polycystic ovaries who are treated in this way become pregnant.

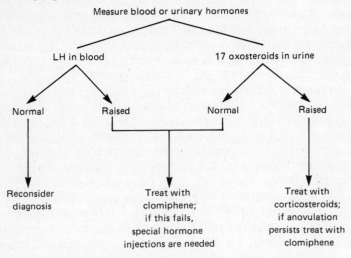

**Figure 2.11**  Principle of treatment of women who have polycystic ovaries and desire pregnancy

## TREATMENT OF DEFECTIVE OVULATION (LUTEAL PHASE DEFICIENCY)

Despite much research the diagnosis and indeed the existence of this condition remains controversial, as does treatment. A variety of hormones have been prescribed and at present some doctors give injections of progesterone in the second half of the menstrual cycle or treat the woman with clomiphene.

## TREATMENT OF PREMATURE OVARIAN FAILURE

Premature ovarian failure is the cause of infertility in 1 per cent of women who have amenorrhea. There are two types of ovarian failure. In the first, the ovary ages prematurely and all the follicles disappear. In other words, the woman reaches the menopause prematurely. In the second type, for some reason, the ovary becomes insensitive to stimulation by the gonadotrophic hormones. Like the Sleeping Beauty it may awaken after a long interval and once again respond to the gonadotrophic hormones, again for no discernible reason. This type of ovarian failure is called the "resistant ovarian syndrome." The two types can be distinguished, in some cases, by analyzing the woman's chromosomes and by taking a small piece of ovarian tissue. If some ovarian follicles are seen when the tissue is examined under a microscope the resistant ovarian syndrome is diagnosed. If no follicles are found the woman has premature ovarian failure; but the examination may miss some follicles, which reduces its accuracy and some specialists say it is invasive and not worth doing.

This poses a problem. How should a woman who desires a pregnancy but may have either the resistant ovarian syndrome or premature ovarian failure be treated? Some women, who presumably have the resistant ovarian syndrome and who are taking hormone replacement treatment for their menopausal symptoms of hot flushes and dry vagina, unexpectedly achieve a pregnancy. But this is uncommon.

Of course, if the woman has premature ovarian failure, an unexpected pregnancy could not happen. Because of the difficulty in making an exact diagnosis, the most effective method of treatment for a woman with premature ovarian failure is for the couple to consider one of the artificial conception techniques (see page 146) using a donor's eggs.

The woman has her uterus prepared to accept an embryo by taking tablets of estradiol and later by the addition of injections or tablets of progesterone. When her hormone levels reach those found after a natural ovulation, the donor's eggs are fertilized by the semen of the woman's husband and are injected, through a laparoscope, into her Fallopian tubes, using the GIFT or ZIFT technique. These techniques have enabled about 50 per cent of women with ovarian failure to become pregnant after one or more attempts.

## TREATMENT OF THYROID PROBLEMS

In about 1 per cent of amenorrheic women, thyroid problems,

usually a deficiency of thyroid hormone, are the cause. Thyroid deficiency responds to treatment with thyroxine.

# SUCCESS RATE FOLLOWING TREATMENT OF OVULATORY DISORDERS

Ovulatory disorders are the cause of infertility in about 20 per cent of couples, They may be associated with other factors, so that the success rate in terms of pregnancy and a 'take home baby' is difficult to determine with accuracy. An attempt has been made in Table 2.1.

**Table 2.1   Success rate of treatment for ovulatory defects, in terms of pregnancies and births (%)**

| Cause | Pregnancy | | Live baby |
|---|---|---|---|
| | No treatment | Drug treatment | |
| Hypothalamic | 30 | 70 | 60 |
| Hyperprolactinaemia | ? | 75 | 65 |
| Defective luteal phase | Unknown | | Unknown |
| Polycystic ovary | ? | 50 | 30 |
| Ovarian failure | 0 | 50 | 40 |

# 3

# Male Factors

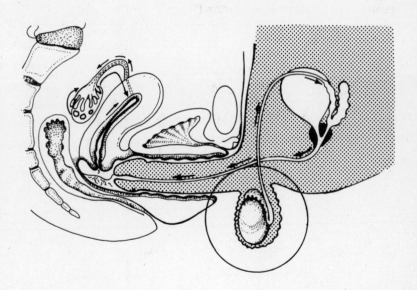

# 3

# Male Factors

Having established, during the interview and history-taking, that the couple have sexual intercourse often enough to expect, by chance or design, that it has occurred during most months at ovulation time, and having found out, by asking the woman, that her partner ejaculates within her vagina, it is usual to arrange to investigate the man. Before discussing this aspect of infertility it may help the reader if something is said about how a man produces sperms.

## THE TESTIS AND SPERM PRODUCTION

The human testis is made up of numbers of long twisting tubules, which join to form larger tubes. (Fig. 3.1a). The tubules make up over 98 per cent of the testicular volume and, at intervals, are separated into compartments by "glistening" tissue. (They look rather like lengths of spaghetti enclosed in the segments of an orange.) The tubules are termed seminiferous tubules because it is here that the sperms are produced. The tubules are supported by connective tissue. Clumps of cells, called Leydig cells, lie in the connective tissue (Fig. 3.1b). Leydig cells play an essential part in the production of sperm.

The seminiferous tubules are lined by germ cells, from which the sperms will develop, going through eight developmental stages, so that the lining in a mature man's testes is eight cells thick. Interspersed between the germ cells are special cells, called Sertoli cells, which have important functions in helping the sperms to mature (Fig. 3.1c). The Sertoli cells nourish the devel-

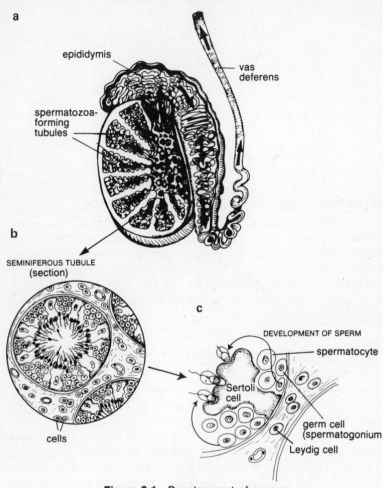

a

epididymis

vas
deferens

spermatozoa-
forming
tubules

b

SEMINIFEROUS TUBULE
(section)

c

DEVELOPMENT OF SPERM

spermatocyte

Sertoli
cell

germ cell
(spermatogonium

Leydig cell

cells

**Figure 3.1** Development of sperms

oping sperms; they remove damaged sperms by absorbing them; they secrete fluid to make a fluid stream, which carries the sperms from the testicular tubules to the epididymis; and they produce the hormone, inhibin, which feeds back to the pituitary and hypothalamus and helps to regulate the release of the gonadotrophic hormones.

With the onset of puberty, the hypothalamus secretes the gonadotrophin-releasing hormone, which induces the pituitary to secrete and release the gonadotrophic hormones into the blood-stream as described in Chapter 2. The hormones, follicle-stimulating hormone (FSH) and the luteinizing hormone (LH), are secreted in both sexes, although in men their names are perhaps misnomers. (Because of this LH is sometimes known as the interstitial-cell-stimulating hormone (ICSH) Fig. 3.2.)

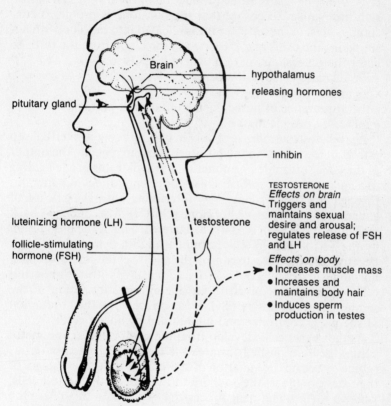

**Figure 3.2**   Control of testicular function and sperm production

FSH circulates in the blood and attaches to "binding sites" on the Leydig cells, which lie in patches between the seminiferous tubules. FSH alters the function of the Leydig cells in some way so that they become receptive to the action of the second gonadotrophic hormone, LH. Released in surges from the pituitary, LH binds on to the surface of the Leydig cells and then enters their substance, where it induces the cells to synthesize and to secrete testosterone. Some of the testosterone rapidly diffuses through the testis, coming into contact with the Sertoli cells in the semi-niferous tubules, which produce a substance that binds the testosterone onto these cells. Testosterone stimulates the adjacent germ cells to develop, through the eight stages, to become sperms. As well, it is now believed that FSH acts directly on the Sertoli cells, inducing testosterone production in them — a sort of fail-safe mechanism to ensure that the hormone is produced constantly. Most of the testosterone is released into the blood-stream supplying the testis and is carried in the blood from the testis to enter the general circulation, where it leads to:

• the increased size of the penis;
• its ability to become erect;
• the appearance of pubic, facial and armpit hair;
• increased muscle mass.

As well, testosterone (probably in part by being converted into estrogen) feeds back to the pituitary gland to regulate the output of the gonadotrophic hormones — a rise in testosterone leading to a fall in gonadotrophins. This action is not direct but operates through the hypothalamus by interfering with the release of gonadotrophin-releasing hormone (GnRH). A second feed-back mechanism has been recently discovered. This is the production by the Sertoli cells of the hormone inhibin, which feeds back negatively to the brain to control the release of the gonadotrophin hormones, particularly FSH. Paradoxically, within the Sertoli cells, inhibin is involved in enhancing the stimulation of the seminiferous tubules by FSH. It can be seen that the production of sperms is controlled and maintained by hormones.

As the sperm cells develop from the germ cells (or spermatogonia) they are pushed towards the center of the seminiferous tubule by the next generation of sperm cells. In the last stages of their development, they adhere to the tips of the Sertoli cells, where a further maturing process takes place. In this phase the sperm cell grows a tail, and the sperm is released to lie free in the cavity of the tubule (Fig. 3.1c). The process of sperm formation takes about 65 days.

Discharged from their nests in the seminiferous tubules the sperms pass along the hollow cavity of the tubule to enter one of the 12 larger connecting tubes. The 12 connecting tubes in turn join to become the twisted convoluted epididymis, and later the vas deferens. The two vas deferens, one from each side, join together in the area of the prostate, and it is here that the sperms are stored prior to ejaculation (Fig. 3.3).

As the sperms pass along the ducts of the epididymis, they

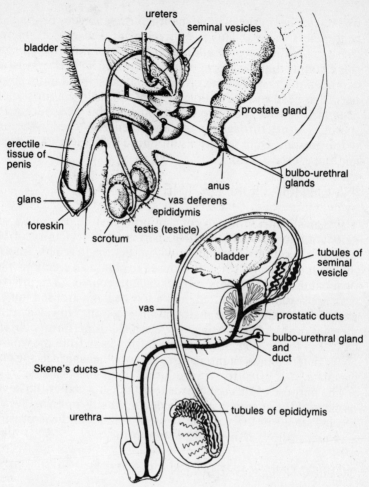

**Figure 3.3** External and internal genital organs of a man

mature further, becoming capable of moving forward as their tails function more effectively. The journey through the epididymis and the vas deferens to the storage area takes about 10 days but is shortened if ejaculation takes place frequently. This means that by the time the sperm is ejaculated it is about 78 days old and has travelled 6 meters (20 ft). In other words, a sperm, which measures 0.005 centimeters has had to journey 120 000 times its own length, the equivalent of a man 1.82 meters (6 ft.) tall swimming 66 kilometers (41 miles). Following ejaculation in a woman's vagina, those sperms that succeed in reaching the ovum, as it lies in the oviduct, have a further journey of about 12 centimeters (6 ins.). This is equivalent to a man, 1.82 meters (6 ft.) tall, swimming 4.5 kilometers (3 miles). It is evident from this example that the sperm requires a great deal of energy to accomplish this task. The energy is created and stored in the lower part of its head and the middle piece of its tail. The nourishment needed to create the energy is probably obtained during the sperm's journey through the vas, and when it is stored in the area of the prostate, from secretions produced by the seminal vesicles and the prostate itself.

# INVESTIGATION OF THE MAN

The man's contribution to conception is that he deposits a sufficient number of live healthy sperms in the vicinity of the woman's cervix by ejaculating within her vagina. This implies that he is sufficiently sexually aroused to obtain an erection of his penis, and is able to take part in sexual intercourse. A few infertile men are sexually unaroused, and a few become aroused but are unable to obtain and to maintain an erection. However, most men in an infertile marriage or relationship perform well sexually. For this reason, after seeking information from the woman about the frequency of intercourse and whether she feels the man ejaculate, it is usual to arrange for a semen analysis.

The purpose of this analysis is to establish whether the development of the sperms has proceeded normally and whether the sperms stored in the vas, the seminal vesicles and the prostate area are healthy, active and not malformed.

## COLLECTING A SPECIMEN OF SEMEN

The man should avoid ejaculating for 2 days before producing the specimen of semen for testing. The reason is that if ejaculation occurs frequently the quantity of the sperms may be reduced. Some laboratories insist that the man attend and masturbate in strange surroundings so that a fresh specimen is obtained, but this is unnecessary and may inhibit or distress the man considerably. It is more pleasant and appropriate for the man to produce the specimen at home. He reaches orgasm either by masturbating or by his partner stimulating his penis, or if the couple prefer by having intercourse and withdrawing before orgasm. This last method is the least preferred as the man has to be fairly agile in withdrawing or he may ejaculate the first part of the semen inside the woman's vagina. As this part of the semen is rich in sperms, the subsequent semen analysis may not be accurate.

The semen should be ejaculated directly into a dry wide-mouthed glass or plastic container. It should not be collected in a condom, as the silicone may damage the sperm, as may a metal container. The container must be dry, as water also interferes with the sperms' activity, tending to immobilize them. The container should be kept at body temperature and should be brought to the laboratory within 2 hours. The couple may observe that the clotted sperm mass liquifies in the container. This is normal.

## THE SEMEN ANALYSIS

The analysis should be made in a laboratory with staff who regularly look at semen, as errors in measurements, and hence in the results, are often large. The following measurements are usually made (see Table 3.1):

**Table 3.1   Criteria for "normal" semen**

| | |
|---|---|
| Volume | — More than 2 ml |
| Sperm count | — More than 20 000 000 per ml |
| Abnormal forms | — *Less* than 40% |
| Motility | — More than 60%, 2 hours after ejaculation |

- The volume of the semen.
- The number of sperms per milliliter.
- The total number of sperms.
- The appearance and shape of a representative number of sperms.
- The percentage of sperms showing good motility after 4 hours.

**Semen volume**   Usually the quantity of semen is more than 2 milliliters — smaller quantities may indicate a problem.

**Sperm concentration**   The number of sperms per milliliter of semen is calculated. The lower limit of "normality" is usually accepted as 20 million per milliliter, but men with lower counts have produced children, so that the lower limit is not an absolute indication of infertility.

**Total number of sperms in the ejaculate**   A total of less than 40 million sperms is usually considered to be "subnormal" although 10 per cent of fertile men have lower total sperm counts.

**Sperm shape and size**   As noted earlier, a normal sperm has an oval head, a short cylindrical body and a long single tail. Abnormal sperms have large heads, or small narrow heads, tapering heads and sometimes double heads or double tails (Fig. 3.4). The number of abnormally shaped or sized sperms in fertile men is very variable but if more than 40 per cent of abnormal forms are found in a specimen of semen, the man's fertility is considered to be impaired. In these cases the man may have varicose veins around his vas deferens. The doctor looks for the condition, known as varicocele, when he examines the man.

**Sperm motility**   The observer notes the number of sperms that are moving progressively forward in a sample of semen examined under a microscope. Sperm motility is obviously an important criterion of the ability of the sperms to fertilize the ovum, as the sperms have to journey through the uterus and oviducts to reach it. Sperm motility is graded, rather subjectively, as: no motility, poor, medium, good or excellent motility. In a normal sample, at least 60 per cent of the sperms examined within 2 hours of ejaculation should show good or excellent forward movement. If no sperms are moving, the condition is called necrospermia. If sperm motility is graded as poor or medium, the condition is called asthenospermia. Diagnosis of necrospermia or asthenospermia is only made after three semen samples are examined. In most cases, asthenospermia is found in association with a low sperm count (oligospermia), but occasionally poor semen motility is found with a normal sperm count.

From this it follows that there are two populations of men who have asthenospermia. The larger group also have oligospermia; the smaller group have a normal sperm count. The two groups may be differentiated by analysing a specimen of the semen, and further information about the man's potential to fertilize his partner's ovum may be obtained by performing a sperm penetration assay (SPA) as described on page 91, where the problems of this test are also discussed.

Some doctors believe that the fertilizing ability of asthenospermic sperms can be enhanced if a course of erythromycin antibiotic is given; however, a carefully controlled study showed that erythromycin was no more beneficial than a placebo.

## Human spermatozoa

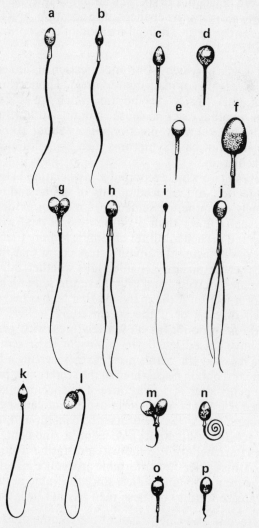

**Figure 3.4**  Normal (a-b) and abnormal (c-p) human sperms: (a) normal;
(b) normal (lateral view); (c) tapering head; (d) pyriform
head; (e) round head; (f) giant head; (g) double head; (h)
double body and tail; (i) pin head; (j) multiple tail; (k)
abnormality of head and body denoting immaturity; (l) bent
body; (m) double head and body abnormality; (n) curled tail;
(o) rough membrane; (p) short tail

The combination of oligospermia and asthenospermia indicates a severe defect of the sperm's ability to fertilize the ovum, considerably reducing the chances of conception, and the couple may consider trying an artificial method of conception, such as GIFT or ZIFT.

**White blood cells in semen**   Chronic infection of the genital tract may follow untreated or inadequately treated gonorrhea or non-gonococcal urethritis (NGU), both of which are sexually transmitted. But in other cases no cause is found. Authorities suggest that "silent" genital tract infection affects about 10 per cent of infertile men; a few have symptoms such as painful urination or painful ejaculation.

Some investigators have reported an association between genital tract infection and reduced quality of semen and because of this routinely examine the semen specimen for evidence of infection. Usually fewer than 5 million leucocytes (white blood cells) are found in each milliliter of semen. If more than 5 million leucocytes are detected the investigators claim that infection is present. Other physicians are uncertain whether infection is a factor in male infertility and only have the semen checked for evidence of infection if the man says that he has had a sexually transmitted disease, or if the sperm count is low. Even this relationship is in doubt, as only a few men with genital tract infection have raised leucocyte counts in their semen. Some physicians massage the man's prostate by inserting a finger into his rectum, and obtain a specimen of the secretion expelled from the man's penis after this procedure. The specimen is then cultured to see if it contains bacteria capable of causing infection and measurements are made of its zinc content and its pH (the degree of acidity or alkalinity). A reduced zinc content and an elevated pH are believed to indicate prostatic infection. Again the value of this rather uncomfortable procedure is in doubt, as is treating the man with antibiotics, since the value of these measures to increase fertility of these men has not been proven.

**Levels of fructose and zinc**   Most of the volume of the semen is provided by secretions from the prostate or the seminal vesicles, sperms only accounting for a small percentage. Some laboratories measure the level of the sugar, fructose, in the specimen although it is known that the value varies very widely in a man's semen at different times. Fructose is secreted by the seminal vesicles, and if it is absent from the specimen, the claim is made that this indicates obstruction to the ducts that lead to the vesicles. How this affects a man's fertility is unknown. Other laboratories measure the level of zinc and a substance called acid phosphatase in the specimen of semen, as these are thought to be indicators of the activity of the prostate in providing nourishment for the sperms. Again it is not known whether correcting abnormal values of zinc improves the man's fertility.

## TWO RARE CONDITIONS THAT CAUSE AZOOSPERMIA

Two rare syndromes account for about 3 per cent of cases of azoospermia in men. The first is called Young's syndrome. The man also has chronic sinusitis and chronic lung infections, with chronic cough and sputum production. The illness is caused by chronic obstruction by thick secretions of the cells lining the epididymis. The disease is slowly progressive and some men have fathered children when younger. Treatment by microsurgery to eliminate the damaged area has not led to pregnancy, although the man's sperm, in his testicle, is normal. A second condition in which the man has enlarged breasts and small testicles (Klinefelter's syndrome) is not amenable to treatment.

## ASSESSMENT OF MALE INFERTILITY

The doctor scrutinizes the results of the semen analysis (see Table 3.1, p. 53) and makes an assessment of the problem. In most cases the lower the sperm count, the higher the proportion of abnormal forms and the poorer the motility of the sperm, but there are exceptions.

The specimen is graded as follows:
• Normal.
• Oligospermia (the sperm count is less than 20 million per milliliter):
— with normally motile sperm,
— with asthenospermia.
• Azoospermia (no sperms seen).
• Asthenospermia, with a normal sperm count.

A normal specimen shows that it is unlikely that the man is "responsible" for the failure of his partner to conceive. An abnormal specimen is an indication to repeat the semen analysis at least twice more, at intervals of 2–4 weeks, before a diagnosis of male sub-fertility or infertility is made, as marked variations in the quality of the semen occur over time and are normal.

During this time the man should be invited to be examined clinically and time provided so that the doctor and the man can talk, since several medical conditions may reduce sperm production.

## CLINICAL ASSESSMENT

If a man is exposed to extremes of heat, to certain chemicals or is taking anti-cancer drugs his sperm count may be low. Some men who are receiving drug treatment for high blood pressure or have diabetes are unable to achieve an erection, others ejaculate into their bladder.

The physical examination of the man is important, particularly examination of his testes and scrotum. The size of his testicles is determined and related to a series of plastic shapes so that the volume of each testis can be judged (Fig. 3.5). Normally the volume of a fertile man's testis is 15 milliliters or greater. The man's scrotum is palpated, particularly where it joins his body, when he is standing. In some cases varicose veins (called a varicocele) can be detected, but in others, they only become recognizable if the man coughs or holds his breath and strains down. For many years it was believed that a varicocele was the cause of a low sperm count, of poor sperm motility, with a large proportion of abnormally shaped sperms in the sample. Several reports indicated that between 15 and 30 per cent of men whose semen analysis showed one or more of these defects had a varicocele, usually on the left side. This opinion can no longer be sustained as recent investigations, using sophisticated techniques, show that varicoceles (both clinically obvious and only detected by special tests such as ultrasound) are found in a similar proportion of men who have a normal sperm count and have fathered children.

This research casts doubt on the claim by many urologists that surgical treatment of the varicocele (by tying the spermatic vein high in the groin) improves the quality of the man's sperms in two-thirds of the men treated. The doubt is increased by reports of carefully designed studies that show no improvement in the quality of the sperms or in pregnancy rates following the operation for varicocele. The conclusion must be that until well designed prospective studies have been made, the operation should no longer be performed.

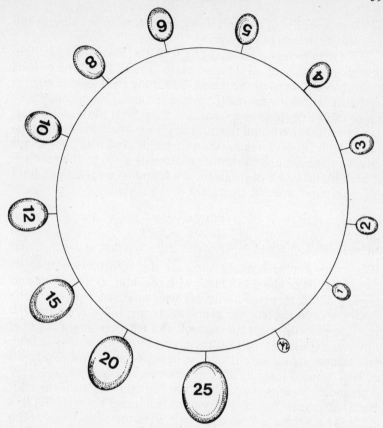

**Figure 3.5** The plastic ellipsoids that comprise the orchidometer; the numbers (marked on the surface of each ellipsoid) indicate volume (ml)

## HORMONE ASSAYS

If the man has azoospermia (in three separate samples of semen) the levels in his blood of the gonadotrophic hormone FSH should be measured. A raised level of FSH (usually three times the expected level) indicates that the man's testicles will not produce sperms, although the production of testosterone by the Leydig cells continues. In other words the man is sterile but virile. This test has replaced a test in which small pieces of testicular tissue were taken (under local anesthesia) for laboratory examination. The biopsy material was examined by a pathologist who looked at the appearance of the cells lining the seminiferous tubules and graded the degree of damage.

If the man has severe oligospermia, that is, fewer than 5 million sperms per milliliter in three separate samples, the level of FSH in his blood should be measured, and if the FSH level is normal and his testicles are normally sized, a testicular biopsy should be made. Some physicians also measure the level of the male hormone, testosterone, and the pituitary hormone, prolactin, in the man's blood as occasionally these are associated with poor sperm counts, although erectile failure is more likely to be the problem if high blood levels of prolactin are found. If a raised prolactin level is found, specific treatment is available.

## THE FINAL ANALYSIS

When the doctor has obtained all the information thought necessary, he or she should talk with the man, at first alone and later, if the man agrees, with his wife or partner present. The doctor should explain the problems in a frank way and give a realistic assessment of the outlook and whether treatment is of any value (Fig. 3.6). By now the man's infertility will have been graded as absolute, severe, relative or unimpaired. *Absolute infertility* is found if the man has azoospermia and raised FSH levels. This indicates testicular failure. On the other hand, if the man has azoospermia but normally sized testes and normal FSH levels, it is likely that a block has occurred in the epididymis or the vas.

*Severe infertility* is diagnosed if the sperm count is less than 5 000 000 per milliliter. Often the man's testicles are small and the level of FSH in his blood is raised. In other cases, the man's testicles are normal size and the FSH level is normal or low. In these cases drugs and hormones are often given to improve the sperm count but the results are poor.

*Relative infertility* is diagnosed if the man's sperm count is between 5 000 000 and 20 000 000 per milliliter, or if there is reduced motility or a large proportion of abnormally shaped sperms. In these cases a varicocele should be looked for, and blood taken to measure the levels of FSH, testosterone and prolactin, although abnormal levels of these last two hormones are not usually found. Treatment may be offered to these men.

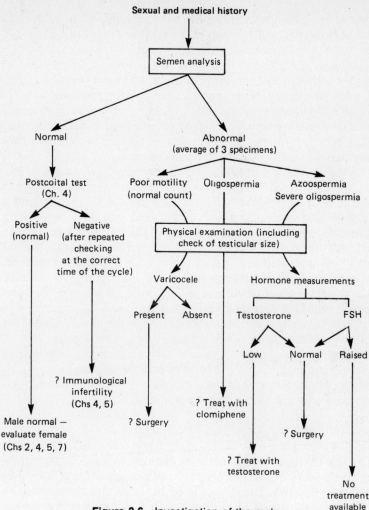

**Figure 3.6** Investigation of the male

# TREATMENT OF MALE INFERTILITY

No current treatment is available for a man who has azoospermia and raised FSH levels in his blood. He is sterile. But if his FSH levels are normal, the azoospermia may be due to a block in the epididymis or the vas, caused by infection. Some microsurgeons

operate to attempt to excise the blocked area and to re-anasto-
mose (join) the healthy parts of the vas; but the results, as far as a
pregnancy is concerned, have been poor.

Men who are found to have *severe infertility* are unlikely to
father a child, although some of them do over a period of time.

Men who have *relative infertility* have a better outlook, as pregnancies do occur without treatment. However, such is the desire
of men who have severe or relative infertility to father a child that
they seek treatment from a variety of sources, both from con-
ventional and from alternative medicine.

A major problem in evaluating the benefits of treatment is that,
as just mentioned, pregnancies occur without treatment. Among
fertile couples pregnancies occur at a rate of 20–30 per cent a
month, and by 1 year about 90 per cent will have achieved a
pregnancy. When the man has relative infertility, the pregnancy
rate falls to about 5–7 per cent a month. Even so, over the period
of a year about 20 per cent of the wives will become pregnant.

A man who is infertile should adopt some general measures.
He should stop smoking and should cease to wear tight underpants. Smoking reduces sperm production and tight underpants
lift up the testicles so that they lie close to the crotch, where the
temperature is raised. This reduces sperm production.

If the man is found to have a varicocele or is diagnosed as
having prostatic infection, surgery may be undertaken or antibiotics given, although, as has been mentioned, the value of each
of these treatments has been questioned.

## DRUG TREATMENT

In the past, many drugs that were thought to improve the quantity or quality of the sperms have been suggested, but none has
proved effective. The drugs listed in Table 3.2 should not be
used. Other drugs, such as mega-vitamin therapy or thyroid hormones, are of no value unless the man is vitamin deficient or has
thyroid disease, both of which are unlikely.

Even treatments that are widely used have not been subjected
to properly designed, scientific trials, which makes the results
reported difficult or impossible to interpret.

It has to be admitted that it is difficult to arrange a controlled
prospective scientific study of the treatment of male infertility.
Two large groups of men with similar semen analysis results
would have to be recruited. One group would be given the "active

**Table 3.2   Drugs of no value in treating male infertility**

Androgens (testosterone)
Tamoxifen (an anti-estrogen)
Erythromycin
Vitamin C
Vitamin E
Caffeine          (suggested as improving
Arginine          sperm motility)
Kallikrein

drug," the other group a placebo. The drug or the placebo would
have to be taken for at least 3 months and follow-up of at least a
year would be needed. Such a trial has not been made, yet on
inadequate evidence, three treatments — testosterone, clomiphene (or one of the other anti-estrogens) and gonadotrophin
therapy — are recommended by some doctors. Is there any
evidence that they are of any value?

## Testosterone therapy

This treatment was introduced in the 1940s, when it was believed
that the male sex hormone would cure a variety of sexual dis-
abilities. The idea was that daily or weekly injections of testosterone would increase the quantity of the sperms in the semen.
After a few years research workers found that testosterone
*decreased* the quantity of sperms, because it suppressed the
release of the gonadotrophic hormones that are necessary for
sperm production. Proponents of testosterone therapy then
changed their ground and argued that when the injections
stopped, a "rebound" surge of gonadotrophin would occur with
increased sperm production, and this might last for up to 2 years.
Doctors who believed in the treatment reported increased sperm
counts and increased pregnancy rates among the patients they
treated, but their reports are difficult to follow, and later studies
have shown no improvement that was not due to chance. In no
case has a properly controlled trial comparing the hormone with
a placebo been made.

Another group of doctors have given a daily dose of an oral
form of testosterone (mesterolone) for a year, and have claimed
improvement in the sperm counts. Once again no control
patients (treated with placebo) were included in the study.

## Anti-estrogens

These substances, of which clomiphene is the most widely known, are used to induce women to ovulate. Clomiphene interferes with the normal "negative" feed-back of the sex hormones, which inhibits the release of gonadotrophic hormones. By blocking the negative feed-back, GnRH is released and in turn induces the pituitary to release FSH and LH. In women this induces ovulation (see p. 37). In men, it was hoped that the same treatment would improve sperm quantity and quality. The drug has to be taken daily (in a dose of 25 milligrams) for at least 3 months, and although improvements in the sperm counts (and some pregnancies) have been reported, they could have occurred by chance. No properly controlled trials of clomiphene have been made.

## Gonadotrophin therapy

In this regimen, the man is given injections of human chorionic gonadotrophin (HCG) in the belief that this will increase the quantity of testosterone *in the testis* and thus improve sperm production. Sometimes the hormone is given in conjunction with human menopausal gonadotrophin (HMG) (HCG is largely LH, and HMG is largely FSH). The hormone is given each day by injection for at least 80 days.

There is no evidence that the injections have any value except in men with severe endocrine disorders.

At present no specific, effective drug treatment is available to improve the sperm count and to increase the chances of a pregnancy. A recent Australian study compared the pregnancy rates of the wives of oligospermic men who had received a variety of treatments. In no instance was drug treatment more effective than no drug treatment.

# INTRAUTERINE INSEMINATION OF "TREATED" HUSBAND'S SEMEN

In this technique the man's semen is concentrated using a complicated laboratory method, the aim of which is to separate the more active sperms from the rest. The man masturbates to produce a sample on the day of his wife's ovulation. The sperms are processed and the more active sperms are introduced into the woman's uterus using the "Tomcat" catheter used in IVF programs.

In the study reported from Adelaide, Australia, men were selected who had at least two of the following: a sperm count of less than 40 million per milliliter; sperm motility of less than 45 per cent; abnormal sperms more than 60 per cent and total sperms in the ejaculate less than 60 million. Using the technique, eight of 39 couples, that is 20 per cent, achieved a pregnancy compared with only one of 34 couples, or 3 per cent, who did not have the treatment. Unfortunately for infertile men subsequent studies of the technique have not been so successful and few pregnancies have occurred. Even if a pregnancy occurs only two-thirds of the women will achieve a "take home baby."

The conclusion must be that intrauterine insemination of treated or untreated husband's semen is not recommended.

## RETROGRADE EJACULATION

A few men reach orgasm but fail to ejaculate because of dysfunction or damage to the internal sphincter of the urethra. This normally closes during ejaculation but in these men it fails to close, permitting the semen to pass backwards into the bladder.

Until recently there has been no effective way of treating this problem, although a few successes have been obtained if the man drinks about a liter of water before sexual intercourse so that his bladder is full. A new technique may be more successful in obtaining sperms so that the couple may achieve a pregnancy. The man takes a teaspoonful of sodium bicarbonate for a few days before masturbating. After reaching orgasm he passes urine into a sterile container. The urine is centrifuged and the sperms are collected. They are treated and the woman is artificially inseminated using the treated sperms.

## ARTIFICIAL CONCEPTION

The recently developed techniques of GIFT, ZIFT and IVF (see Chapter 8) are now being used to treat men who have oligospermia or azoospermia. These techniques obviate the need for the sperms to make the journey through the woman's genital tract and may enable fresher sperms to fertilize the egg. Early reports show that the techniques have achieved some pregnancies but more work is needed before their place can be determined.

This comment also applies to a new technique in which a single sperm is 'microinjected' through the zona pellucida of eggs obtained by the IVF technique. The technique may help men who are severely oligospermic or asthenospermic. A few pregnancies using the technique have been reported. More research is required to determine its value.

# PSYCHOLOGICAL EFFECT OF MALE INFERTILITY

In our culture men are expected not only to be potent and to take the initiative in sexual encounters, but are expected to be fertile. It is only in the past 50 years that the contribution of men to infertility has been recognized. Before that time, infertility was blamed on women.

Clearly, the diagnosis by a doctor that a man has absolute or relative infertility may have considerable psychological consequences, and the man usually goes through the phase of grief, described on page 109. The impact of the knowledge that the infertility may be attributed to him can be reduced if the doctor is sympathetic and understanding. An offhand, authoritarian manner may be most damaging to the man. For example, if the diagnosis is that of absolute infertility — in other words that the man is sterile — the information should be given to him in person. The doctor should never give the bad news by phone. It is cruel and may be destructive to the man's feeling of worth. The information should only be given directly during a visit and the man must be allowed time to discuss the problem, time to adjust and the opportunity to discuss the options available.

If the couple trust the doctor and are able to talk with him or her, the psychological damage of male sterility is minimized.

# SEXUAL DYSFUNCTION AS A CAUSE OF INFERTILITY

A small number of men, who attend with their wife or partner because of continuing infertility, are found either to have a low level of sexual desire or of sexual arousal or to have erectile failure. A low level of sexual desire limits the frequency of sexual intercourse; erectile failure (also called impotence) prevents intra-vaginal ejaculation of sperms.

Although these factors are uncommon causes of infertility, a couple seeking help must be comfortable about answering questions regarding their sexual relationships and their sexual activity.

There are many causes of reduced sexual desire and arousal and of erectile failure. Reduced sexual desire usually has a psychological cause. Erectile failure is due to illness in about half of the cases and has a psychological origin in the other half (Tables 3.3 and 3.4). Once physical causes have been eliminated, sexual counselling will help to resolve the problem.

**Table 3.3   Main factors involved in erectile failure in men investigated for infertility**

| | |
|---|---|
| • Physical: | |
|     Diabetes | |
|     Alcoholism (liver disease) | |
|     Neurological disease, e.g. multiple sclerosis | |
|     Hypothyroidism | 50% |
| • Following drugs: | |
|     Antihypertensive drugs | |
|     Some antidepressants | |
|     Some tranquillizers | |
| • Psychological: | |
|     Depression (as a cause or as an effect) | |
|     Marital discord | 50% |
|     "Performance anxiety" | |
|     Fear of failure | |

**Table 3.4   Factors involved in reduced (inhibited) sexual desire or arousal**

- Strict "religious" upbringing, in which sexuality was either not discussed or was considered "dirty"
- Poor relationship with partner
- Illness, either physical or psychological, especially depression

# 4

# The "Cervical Factor" and the Postcoital Test

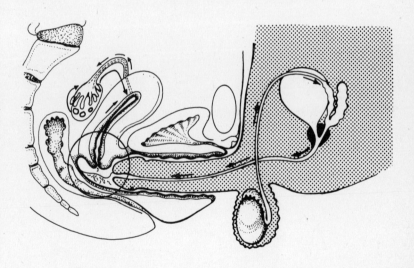

# 4

# The "Cervical Factor" and the Postcoital Test

In order to enter the uterus, the ejaculated sperms have to travel through the twisting channels in the mucus secreted by the cells that line the cervical canal. This is only possible at certain times during the menstrual cycle, as the character of the mucus depends on the level of estrogen in the blood. As the level of estrogen rises to a peak just before ovulation (Fig. 4.1), the quantity of mucus secreted increases (Fig. 4.2), and its character changes from being thick, sticky, matted and cloudy to becoming clear, elastic and stretchable. It also forms long threads, which separate, creating channels in the cervical mucus (Fig. 4.3). These changes are most pronounced at the time of ovulation. Two days after ovulation, the quantity of mucus has diminished considerably, and it has become sticky and relatively impervious to sperms once again because of the influence of progesterone, which is now being secreted by the ovary.

You can understand from this that for most of the menstrual cycle the mucus is largely impenetrable, and it is only when the channels form during the days around ovulation that sperms can readily reach the uterine cavity and beyond. The observation that poor sperm penetration of cervical mucus might be a factor in infertility occurred as long ago as 1866. Dr. Marion Sims, an American gynecologist, suggested that if a specimen of cervical mucus was obtained a few hours after intercourse, and examined for the presence or absence of sperms, a greater insight into infertility might be obtained. However, the prevailing medical and social ethics prevented him from exploring the idea. In 1913, another American gynecologist, Max Huhner, revived the idea and the "cervix test," or postcoital test, was established.

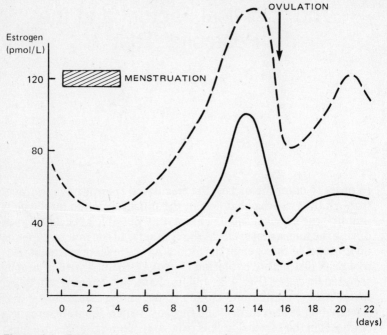

**Figure 4.1**  Estrogen levels during the menstrual cycle (range: dotted lines)

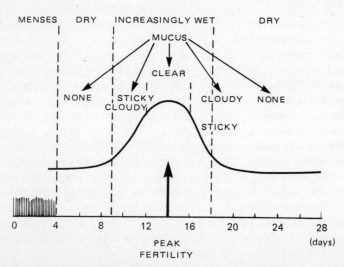

**Figure 4.2**  The menstrual cycle and cervical mucus

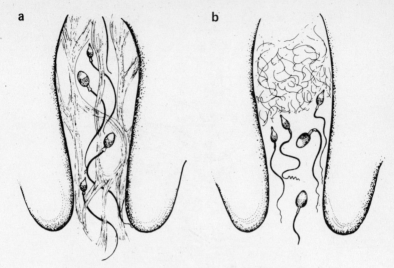

**Figure 4.3**  (a) Cervical mucus at ovulation time
(b) at other times of the menstrual cycle

# THE POSTCOITAL TEST

In the past 70 years the test has been performed during the investigation of large numbers of infertile couples, often repeatedly
but with little agreement on the way it is to be performed or in the
manner of evaluating the findings. The few objective evaluations
have been adversely criticized by proponents and opponents of
the test, often more emotionally than rationally.

In brief, the test is made in the following way. The couple have
sexual intercourse on one of the 2 days before ovulation or on the
day of ovulation. The man ejaculates, and later withdraws his
penis from the woman's vagina. She lies on her back for 20
minutes and then, at a time decided by her doctor, usually 8–12
hours later, attends his office, so that a specimen of her cervical
mucus (with the sperm contained in it) may be removed from her
cervix (Fig. 4.4). This is usually done by inserting a narrow plastic
tube into the cervix, attaching it to a syringe and drawing some of
the mucus into the tube, which is then clipped. The sample is
placed on a slide and examined under a microscope, or is examined directly in the plastic tube that was inserted into the cervix
to take the specimen.

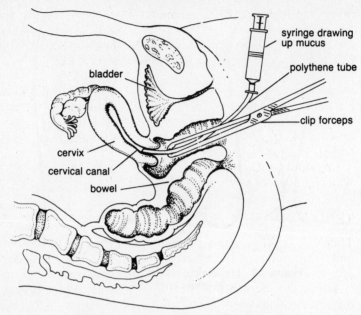

**Figure 4.4** Sampling cervical mucus

## RATIONALE OF THE POSTCOITAL TEST

Initially the test was used to confirm that the man had ejaculated sperm into the woman's vagina. At that time it was considered improper or immoral to ask a man to practice withdrawal or to masturbate to produce a specimen of his semen. It is now known that the *quality* of the man's semen cannot be determined from the postcoital test and that a semen analysis is essential for this purpose, so that the use of the postcoital test for this reason has been superseded.

A few predominantly chauvinistic gynecologists continue to use the test to *prove* that the man has ejaculated within the woman's vagina, believing that some women are unable to identify that this has occurred during sexual intercourse, or are unable to detect when the semen seeps out of the vagina after withdrawal of the man's penis.

The majority of gynecologists who use the postcoital test do so to determine whether the ejaculated sperms are able or are unable to penetrate the cervical mucus at the time of ovulation. Lack of penetration may be due to one of two causes, the first being that there is no cervical mucus, and second that for some reason, probably immunological, the ability of the sperms to penetrate the mucus is impaired — in other words sperm function is defective. In this case the problem is more likely to be with the man rather than the woman.

The first cause is uncommon and is only likely if the woman has had an operation on her cervix that has eliminated the glands lining the cervical canal, or if it has been treated too aggressively by cautery, by freezing or by laser to cure abnormal cervical cells.

Impaired sperm function is looked for in several further tests, which are described in the next chapter.

## TECHNIQUE OF THE POSTCOITAL TEST

The PCT is only helpful if the technique for its use is adhered to, and if the test is sensitive enough to detect what it is claimed to be able to detect. To achieve this, three criteria must be met.

The first criterion is that the test must be made on one of the 2 days before ovulation or on the day of ovulation. The second criterion is that the man should have avoided ejaculating for 2 days before the test. The third criterion is that the woman should lie on her back for 20 minutes after the man has ejaculated in her vagina.

Two clinical and one laboratory method are available to meet the first criterion. The clinical methods are: (1) to examine a sample of the cervical mucus each day around the time of ovulation to determine its quantity, its stretchability and its appearance; (2) to study the woman's basal body temperature chart.

The first test depends on the fact that the character of the cervical mucus is determined by the level of estrogen in the body. During the first half of the menstrual cycle the level of estrogen rises, peaking about 2 days before ovulation. As described earlier, influenced by the rising estrogen levels, the cervical mucus alters in character. About 4 days before ovulation, the mucus increases in quantity, becomes clear in appearance and is stretchable. The ability of the mucus to stretch can be tested if a drop is placed on a slide and is drawn up using a surgical forceps (Fig. 4.5). Another way is to place a drop on the thumb, put the forefinger on the drop and separate the thumb and forefinger to see how far the mucus stretches without breaking. The changes reach their peak in the 24 hours before and after ovulation. A further change

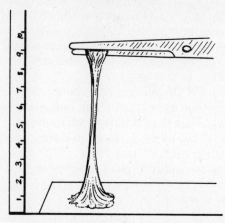

**Figure 4.5**  Cervical mucus. Testing for spinnbarkeit or stretchability

occurs to the mucus at the time of ovulation. If a sample is looked at through a microscope before ovulation, it looks like a smudge; at ovulation the smudge changes into a pattern resembling a fern (Fig. 4.6).

The second clinical test depends on the observation that a woman's basal body temperature (that is her temperature taken when she is resting, just after waking up) falls just before ovulation and then rises.

The laboratory test was introduced when doctors found that basal body temperature charting was rather inaccurate. The test

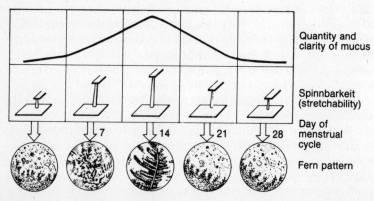

**Figure 4.6**  Changes in the cervical mucus during a menstrual cycle

measures the level of luteinizing hormone (LH) in the woman's saliva or blood daily for about 4 days before the expected day of ovulation. The level suddenly doubles about 30–36 hours before ovulation.

## Problems with the PCT

Some investigators who use the PCT have failed to recall that the cervical mucus is only receptive to sperm in the 2 days before ovulation. By failing to meet the first of the criteria they have concluded that the cause of infertility was the "cervical factor" when they took the sample on an inappropriate day.

The second problem is that there is no agreement how long after ejaculation the sample should be taken and examined through a microscope. The length of time after ejaculation affects the number of "actively forward-moving sperms." Some experts take the sample from the woman's cervix 2 hours after intercourse, others suggest waiting for 24 hours. Probably the most informative time gap between intercourse and taking the sample is 8–12 hours, as the sample taken during this period may more readily suggest that an immunological problem is present and is affecting sperm penetration of the cervical mucus.

## INTERPRETATION OF THE POSTCOITAL TEST

There are no consistent criteria that are accepted for interpreting the test. Some investigators insist that the test is negative unless 10 or more sperms, moving forwards, are seen in each field examined with the high-power lens of the microscope. Others demand 20 or more actively progressing sperms per high-power field before they call the test positive. Other investigators claim that if only a few sperms with "directional motility" are seen the test is positive. Still others say that the test is positive if five or fewer motile sperms are seen in the mucus.

A problem of accepting any of these criteria is that pregnancies occur frequently to women who have a negative postcoital test. While it is possible that, in these women, the postcoital test was made on an inappropriate day, it may indicate that the test has limited value. For example, a group of women whose postcoital test was negative were examined on the same day by laparoscopy and in most of them sperms were recovered from the peritoneal cavity. It is also clear that the actual number of sperms found "progressing" in the mucus correlates poorly with subsequent pregnancies. This has led one group of investigators to conclude: "Our results are based only on the presence of spermatozoa in the mucus and whether they are showing active progression or not."

A second group of researchers concluded: "Any postcoital analysis which shows *any* motile spermatozoa should be considered as indicating a normal result." A third group of investigators have written that "A negative test has little clinical value and must be repeated."

## *IN-VITRO* TESTS

A number of doctors, particularly if they are engaged in infertility research, use *in-vitro* tests to detect sperm penetration of cervical mucus. The tests are also used by some when a negative postcoital test has been found. Two tests are used currently. These are the slide test, and the capillary penetrability test.

### THE SLIDE TEST

A drop of cervical mucus (taken at ovulation time and checked for clarity and stretchability) is placed on a microscope slide and covered with a thin glass coverslip. A drop of freshly produced

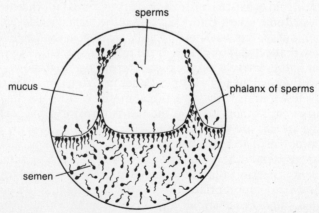

**Figure 4.7**   The slide–mucus sperm penetration test, as viewed through a microscope

semen is placed at the edge of the coverslip. The semen is drawn under the coverslip by capillary action and makes contact with the cervical mucus. Examination of the slide under a microscope (sometimes after incubating it at 37°C for 30 minutes) shows an interface between the semen and the mucus. Active sperm invasion across the interface indicates that there is no hostility between the cervical mucus and the sperms (Fig. 4.7). Although the test is simple to perform, it is not easily quantifiable and is difficult to reproduce, which diminishes its value.

## THE CAPILLARY PENETRABILITY TEST

A Dutch doctor has invented an apparatus that he claims closely imitates conditions in the cervical canal and that he uses for testing the sperm's ability to penetrate cervical mucus. The apparatus consists of a flat tube with a small reservoir at one end (Fig. 4.8). Cervical mucus is drawn into the tube directly from the cervix and one end is then sealed. The other end is placed in the reservoir into which a sample of the man's sperms has been placed. The apparatus is put in an incubator at 37°C for 2 hours, and the movement of the sperms through the mucus is observed by looking at the tube through a microscope at the end of the incubation period. The distance the sperms have travelled, their number at each distance, and how long they remain motile is recorded.

## HOW CAN THIS INFORMATION BE INTERPRETED?

The most that can be said is that a positive postcoital test indicates that there is no immunological barrier to infertility in either the man's sperm or the woman's cervical mucus. A negative test performed in the 2 days before or on the day of ovulation merely indicates that there may be an immunological or a sperm factor that is hindering or preventing conception. If the test is not performed at the time of ovulation it indicates only that the doctor has wasted his and his patient's time. Before any further testing is considered the doctor should recheck the man's semen analysis (which should have been made previously), as a low sperm count, or a high proportion of abnormal sperms in the specimen, are known to be associated with poor or absent sperm penetration of cervical mucus.

Once the quality of the man's semen is assured the couple should be offered one of the choices by which the cervical mucus

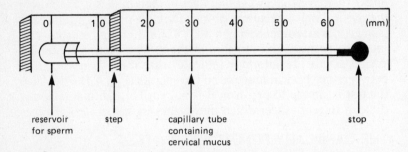

**Figure 4.8**  Capillary sperm penetration test (viewed through a
microscope, sperms' penetration of more than 20 mm
shows that no abnormality is present)

can be investigated. These are to: (1) repeat the test, perhaps on
several occasions; (2) perform an *in-vitro* sperm penetrability
test; or (3) investigate the couple for serum or cervical antibodies,
as discussed in Chapter 5 (see Fig. 4.9).

Discussion with the couple is important, as the first choice,
that of repeating the postcoital test, may be inappropriate for
some women whose psychosexual relationships may deteriorate
unless the purpose, the imperfections and the lack of reliability of
the test are explained. On the other hand a positive test has a
beneficial psychological and physiological effect, as the couple
can be told that it is extremely unlikely that any sperm defect or
immunological factors that might interfere with conception are
present. In *the absence* of any other cause for infertility, a positive
postcoital test is associated with a fourfold higher pregnancy rate,
in the next 3 years, than a negative test.

## POOR SPERM FUNCTION

Until recently most investigators have believed that the poor
quality of cervical mucus was the cause of the infertility as
sperms were unable to negotiate its twisting channels to reach the
cavity of the uterus. This belief may have been wrong, at least in
some cases. Studies in Bristol, England, suggest that a negative
postcoital test may indicate that the sperm's penetration function is defective, even when the sperm analysis is normal. In the
study the doctors investigated the ability of sperms to fertilize

CRITERIA

- The test must be performed on one of the 2 days before, or on, the day of ovulation

- The semen analysis results must be available

- The test is made 6–12 hours after sexual intercourse

- At least five sperms, actively moving forward, are seen under the microscope in each 'high-power field' for the test to be designated positive

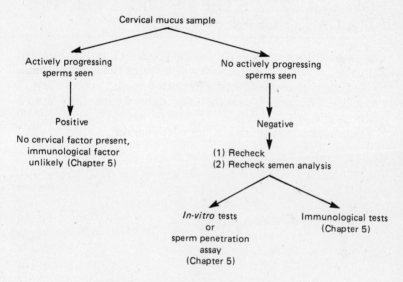

**Figure 4.9**   The postcoital test: action chart

human eggs (in the manner of the IVF program). Three infertile groups of women were chosen: (1) women with tubal damage; (2) couples with a negative PCT; (3) couples whose infertility was unexplained after full investigation. The fertilization rate in couples where the women had tubal damage was 80 per cent, and in couples with unexplained infertility but a normal, positive PCT it was 68 per cent. In couples with a negative PCT or unexplained infertility and a negative PCT, only 16 per cent and 36 per cent of the eggs were fertilized.

The above findings suggest that a negative PCT indicates in many cases that the sperm's ability to fertilize the egg is defective, rather than it being unable to penetrate the cervical mucus. In a few cases, it may also indicate an immunological reason for the infertility.

The investigation of defective sperm function using the IVF techniques poses ethical problems. Is it ethical to obtain human eggs and attempt to fertilize them to obtain a diagnosis or must the test be followed by replacement of the embryo in the mother's uterus?

## HOW COMMON IS THE CERVICAL FACTOR AS A CAUSE OF INFERTILITY

The intensity with which the investigations should be pursued has to be related to the frequency with which the cervical factor or the defective sperm function factor is believed to be a cause of infertility. The consensus is that it accounts for between 2 and 5 per cent of cases at most.

Treatment is considered in the next chapter.

# 5
# Immunological Factors

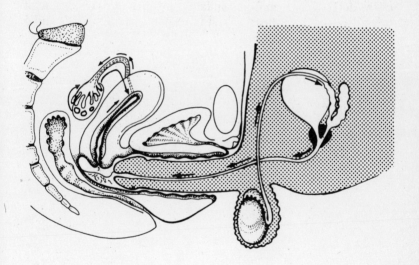

# 5

# Immunological Factors

There are claims that immunological factors are a cause of infertility in between 1 and 3 per cent of infertile couples. Investigation of these factors using laboratory tests has stirred the minds (and sometimes the imaginations) of many investigators, with the result that a large number of tests have been devised. Many of these tests, which purported to give accurate estimations of the extent of the problem, have been shown to be inaccurate, and are of little help, often confusing rather than clarifying the problem. The more recent tests are more specific. Despite the laboratory advances in the investigation of the immunology of infertility, it is still not certain that immunological factors are really causes of infertility, and treatment is both non-specific and disappointing.

To understand the background it is appropriate to consider, briefly, the basis of the immunological reaction in humans.

## HUMAN IMMUNOLOGY

A feature of some of the cells that make up the human body is that they are able to distinguish between cells that are derived from the fertilized egg, which divided again and again and differentiated to make the body, and cells from other organisms. In other words the body distinguishes the self and the non-self. It is able to identify non-self tissues, cells, proteins and other large molecules and is able to separate them into harmless non-self cells and potentially harmful cells. Having made this distinction it either ignores them (in the first case) or defends the body against them (in the second case).

Those cells in the human body that possess the power to distinguish the harmless and potentially harmful non-self cells that get into the body, and then are able to attack the harmful non-self cells, constitute the body's immune system. Occasionally, the cells of the body's immune system fail to recognize that a cell is self, and produce substances that attack it, leading to auto-immune disease. But in most cases only non-self cells are identified and attacked.

When a potentially harmful cell, that is one that the person's immune system "perceives" as harmful, is detected a complex series of events occurs.

On the surface of the non-self cell there are specialized patches of molecules called antigens, which provoke the immune system to respond. When the foreign cell, with the specifically shaped antigen sites on its surface, first enters the body, it provokes a reaction to the invasion (Fig. 5.1). The first cells of the immune system that reach the foreign cells are called T4 helper lympho-cytes (Fig. 5.1). (They are called T cells to recognize their origin in the thymus gland.) Abundant numbers of T4 lymphocytes circulate in the blood and in the lymphatic system and they are also found in considerable quantities in the liver, the spleen and the lungs. Specialized groups (clones) of cells are programmed to recognize antigen sites on the surface of foreign cells and are attracted to these cells. The programmed T4 cells divide repeatedly to produce a group of identical cell clones. The clones produce substances called lymphokines, which enter the blood. The lymphokines have several functions. First, they transform the programmed T4 cells to make clones of cells called T8 cytotoxic (killer) cells. The T8 cells have areas on their surface indentical in shape to those of the antigen sites on the foreign cells. When the two areas come into contact they interlock or bind. Second, the T8 cells activate other lymphocytes, called macrophages, to surround and destroy the foreign cells. Third, and most importantly, they induce another type of lymphocyte called B cells (because they are formed in the bone marrow) to produce antibodies, specific for each foreign cell's antigens. Once formed the antibodies circulate in the blood for months or years, either because further "invasions" of identical antigens enter the body, which starts the formation of antibodies again, or because the cells are able to pass on to their descendants the ability to make antibodies to a specific antigen. Eight classes of antibody have been identified. One of these is the most common antibody and is called immu-

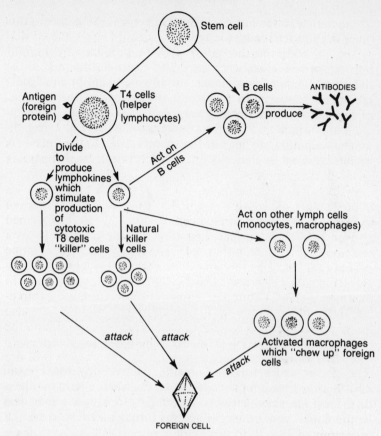

**Figure 5.1** Diagram representing the body's response to the presence of a "harmful" cell, with antigens on its surface

noglobulin G (IgG). Another is immunoglobulin A (IgA), which is secreted by the cells that line body cavities, such as the cells of the cervix, as well as circulating in the blood. IgA is probably the most important antibody in infertility.

# THE IMMUNOLOGY OF INFERTILITY

In a few cases of infertility it is believed that the immune system of the man or the woman is provoked to produce antibodies to sperms. The antibodies then prevent the sperms from migrating through the cervical canal, effectively preventing them from reaching and fertilizing the egg.

The antibodies to the sperms may be produced by the man himself, in which case they are called "auto-antibodies," or by the woman. In the first instance, the antisperm antibodies "coat" the tail of the sperm. In the second, the antibodies coat the head of the sperm. When the affected sperms are ejaculated into the woman's vagina and begin to penetrate the cervical canal, the antibody coat on the head of the sperms sticks to the threads of mucus secreted by the cells lining the cervical canal (Fig. 5.2).

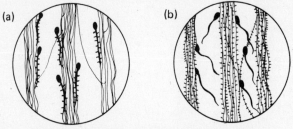

**Figure 5.2**  Sperm immobilization (the shaking phenomenon):
(a) antibodies in the male — the sperm tails coated with antibodies stick to the strands of cervical mucus;
(b) antibodies in the female — the sperm heads stick to the mucus

The sperms are immobilized, unable to move forwards. The tail continues to thrash for a while so that the whole sperm oscillates or shakes. The shaking can be detected by looking at a specimen of the mucus containing the sperms through a microscope.

## IMMUNOLOGICAL TESTS

### Agglutination tests

In most cases of immunological infertility, the antisperm antibodies are produced by the woman in her blood and seep through the cells of her cervical canal. When they come into contact with the ejaculated sperms they cause them to clump or agglutinate (Fig. 5.3). The sperm agglutination can be detected by mixing a sample of the man's sperm with a sample of the woman's blood serum on a slide or in a test-tube. This test has recently been found not to be specific for sperm antibodies, as sperms may be agglutinated by some chemicals and, occasionally, when a pregnant woman's blood serum is added to her husband's sperm! Because of this non-specificity most scientists have abandoned

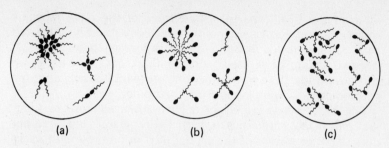

**Figure 5.3**  Sperm microagglutination patterns: (a) head-to-head;
(b) tail-to-tail; (c) head-to-tail

the tube–slide sperm agglutination test, and a similar "tray agglutination" test.

## Sperm immobilization test

To overcome the problem of non-specificity new tests have been developed. The first is the sperm immobilization test. The test attempts to find out if either partner's blood contains antibodies that may immobilize sperm. A sample of the man's blood serum is added to a sample of the semen of a fertile man. In another test-tube a sample of the woman's blood serum is added to a sample of the same fertile man's semen. A control tube is also set up. This contains serum and semen from fertile donors. A substance called complement is added to the three tubes and they are incubated for 60 minutes. The percentage of mobile sperms is counted in each of the tubes, and the ratio between the mobile proportion in each of the tested specimens and those in the control tube is calculated. If two or more times the number of sperms have been immobilized in either of the tested specimens compared with the control, the test is positive and an immunological problem, which may be the cause of the infertility, is presumed to exist.

## Radioimmunoassay of IgG

Another method of detecting immunological infertility is to measure the level of antisperm antibody (immunoglobulin IgG) in the blood serum of both partners of a couple who have unexplained infertility. Using a sophisticated radioimmunoassay, out of 514 infertile American couples, 7 per cent of the men and 13 per cent of the women were found to have IgG antisperm antibodies in their blood. The scientists followed six couples in which three of the female partners and three of the male partners showed the antibodies. Four of the affected partners were treated with corticosteroids (see p. 94) and two pregnancies resulted. The two remaining affected people, both women, were not given corticosteroids. Both women became pregnant but only after the antibodies had disappeared from their blood.

The three tests described above have two disadvantages. First, they only detect antibodies to sperm in the person's blood, rather than in the secretions of the genital tract or on the sperm itself. Second, they give no indication of the type of antibody present.

## Sperm cervical mucus contact test (SCMC)

More information may be obtained from a test called the "sperm cervical mucus contact test" (SCMC). In this test a sample of mucus from the woman's cervix is mixed with a sample of her husband's sperms on the slide, or in a tube. It is also mixed on another slide with a sample of sperms from a fertile man (who has no antisperm antibodies in his serum). In other tubes or slides, samples of the husband's sperms and the donor's sperms are mixed with samples of mucus from a known fertile woman's cervical mucus. The samples are examined under a microscope. The test is shown diagramatically as follows:.

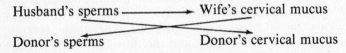

The test is interpreted in the following manner. It is considered positive if sperms are seen moving forward though the cervical mucus and negative if they are immobile or shaking. Using the SCMC test it can be determined whether the husband's sperms carry the antibodies, in which case they will be immobilized by the wife's cervical mucus and by the donor's cervical mucus. If the wife's cervical mucus also immobilizes the husband's and donor's sperms, it is likely that she is producing antibodies against all sperms.

## The immunobead test

This recently developed test may supersede the other tests described. Microscopic polyacrylamide beads are coated with rabbit antihuman immunoglobulin G or immunoglobulin A. The beads are added to a sample of sperms. If the sperms have antigen sites on their surface, the beads will stick to them. The sample is examined under a microscope and the number of sperms that have immunobeads attached are counted. If more than half of the sperms have immunobeads attached the test is regarded as positive (Fig. 5.4).

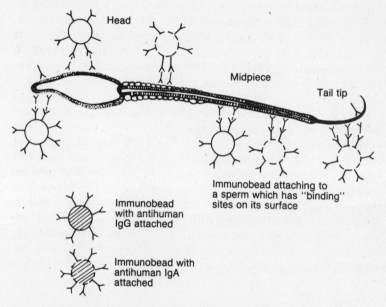

Immunobead attaching to a sperm which has "binding" sites on its surface

Immunobead with antihuman IgG attached

Immunobead with antihuman IgA attached

**Figure 5.4**  Diagrammatic representation of sperm antibodies coating sperm surface and immunobead binding

## SPERM PENETRATION ASSAY (SPA)

The problem with the tests already discussed is that neither the postcoital test nor the immunological tests can differentiate men whose sperms are unable to fertilize an ovum from those whose sperms may do so after an interval of months or years. Even if the sperms are able to reach the ovum they may not be able to penetrate the zona pellucida and fertilize it. This suggested to a Japanese scientist in 1976 that it might be useful to observe the process of fertilization. On ethical and moral grounds it is impossible to use human ova, so he decided to use hamster's eggs. Hamsters are cheap, breed rapidly, are easy to care for and readily available. The chosen animal is induced to superovulate by giving it injections of gonadotrophins (in the same way that anovulatory women are induced to ovulate). About 72 hours after the first injection the animal is killed, and the eggs "harvested." The zona pellucida of each egg is stripped chemically so that only the ovum remains. Each naked ovum is placed on a microscope slide in contact with a droplet of the man's semen, which has been incubated in a special solution to achieve capacitation. The slide is incubated for about 3 hours and the percentage of hamster's eggs containing swollen sperm heads is counted. Men who have fathered children have an average score of 50 per cent, meaning that half of the eggs counted contain swollen sperm heads. However, the range for fertile men is very wide, ranging from 10 per cent to 90 per cent. The research suggests that if the score is less than 15 per cent, the man is unlikely to father a child, but this is disputed.

This test is still under study as there are many factors that render its results invalid. First, the wide range of positive tests found in fertile men. Second, the type of solution in which the sperms are incubated makes a difference, as does the duration of the incubation. Third, there is little standardization between laboratories. In 1988, two American scientists reviewed the world literature about the test and came to the conclusion that "until the validity and reproducibility of the sperm penetration assay have been established, this expensive test should probably not be used to evaluate infertile couples."

# TREATMENT

The detection of sperm antibodies in the blood serum of one or both partners of an infertile marriage, or the finding of a positive immunobead test has led doctors to suggest five different treatments, which, it is claimed, may help the couple achieve a pregnancy.

1   The first and oldest method is to prevent sperms from coming into contact with the woman's tissues. The man uses a condom each time he has sexual intercourse and the couple avoid oral sex.

The theory behind this treatment is that in the absence of a continuing stimulus, in the form of sperms, the woman's immunocompetent cells cease to produce any antisperm antibodies and their concentration in the blood drops to very low levels.

2   The second method is to treat the partner who has the anti-sperm antibodies with corticosteroids. Corticosteroids act by inhibiting the body's immune cells from making antibody, and the serum level of the antibodies falls. Both high and low doses of corticosteroids have been tried.

3   The third method is to use the husband's semen and to inject it into the uterine cavity at the time the woman is ovulating. This is known as artificial insemination of husband's semen (AIH).

4   The fourth method, which is rather more sophisticated than the third, depends on the hypothesis that antisperm antibodies in the man's blood seep into his prostate area, where the sperms collect, and enter the seminal fluid. The antibodies fix onto the sperm antigens. When the ejaculated sperms try to penetrate the spiral channels in the cervical mucus, the antibody–antigen complexes are activated and act like hooks. These attach the sperms to the strands of cervical mucus. Scientists who believe in this theory suggest that the complexes can be removed if the man ejaculates into a special solution (Tyrode's solution), which is then centrifuged. The sperms migrate to the end of the tube. The liquid at the top of the centrifuge tube is discarded and the sperms are resuspended in Tyrode's solution. This is referred to as "washing." Two further washings are carried out, and the washed sperms are injected into the woman's uterus at ovulation time.

5   The fifth method is to determine when the woman is about to ovulate, by examining her ovaries with ultrasound each day. At the time of ovulation, a narrow flexible tube is threaded through the uterine cavity and along the Fallopian tube on the side of the ovary that is about to ovulate. Sperms are then injected along the tube.

## HOW SUCCESSFUL IS TREATMENT?

Success has been reported when each of these methods has been used, but studies in which some patients have been given treatment while others have received no treatment showed that the same proportion of couples became pregnant in each group.

Following the use of condoms for 6 months and then regular intercourse, about 30 per cent of the women became pregnant within a year, which is about the same proportion of pregnancies among couples with immunological infertility who did not use condoms.

The success rate following AIH is lower, only 20 per cent of women achieving a pregnancy. The probable reason for this is that if an immunological problem is present, immunological factors may interfere with the passage of the sperms through the Fallopian tube.

The results of sperm washing and intra-uterine insemination have been poorly reported, but a few pregnancies have been claimed to be due to the use of this technique.

The benefit of high-dose corticosteroid treatment is also hard to evaluate, as most reports are about patients whose sperm antibodies were identified by methods now considered inaccurate. Unless the antibodies are attached to the sperm itself, sperm antibodies in blood are probably unimportant. A recent double-blind controlled trial avoided these methodological problems. Twenty-four men were treated with corticosteroids and were compared with 19 men who were not treated. Corticosteroids or placebo were given for 7 days each month for 3 months. At the end of this time 3 (12 per cent) of the wives of the treated men had become pregnant, as had 1 wife (5 per cent) of the untreated men, results that are not statistically different.

High-dose corticosteroid treatment is not without danger. Six per cent of men treated may vomit blood or develop damage to the head of the thigh bone (femoral head avascular necrosis). About 20 per cent of men treated develop indigestion, hip pain, aggressive behavior or visual disturbances. High-dose corticosteroid treatment should never be recommended unless the man is aware of the hazards.

Recently, low-dose corticosteroids (prednisolone, 20 mg twice daily), taken with meals by the man each day for the first 10–12 days of the woman's menstrual cycle, have been tried, with some success (compared with a placebo), and no serious side-effects.

It is possible that the new reproductive technologies, GIFT, ZIFT and IVF or the injection of selected sperms into the outer end of the Fallopian tube, may improve the pregnancy rate in cases of immunological infertility. These techniques avoid the need for sperms to "swim" through the woman's genital tract and would avoid the effect of antisperm antibodies on their forward progression.

It will be clear from this discussion that the concept of an immunological cause for infertility and the investigations to establish that it exists pose several problems. The first is that many of the tests are not specific. The second is that few properly controlled, well designed clinical trials have been conducted.

Perhaps the main benefit of making the tests is to reassure the couple that they do not have a supposed immunological cause for their infertility.

# SEX PRESELECTION

It is well established that the sex of the child is determined by the male sperm. Each ovum contains in its nucleus 23 chromosomes, one of which is the sex chromosome X, so called because of its shape. In contrast, there are two populations of sperms, which exist in about equal numbers in the man's ejaculate. One population has a chromosomal content of 23, one of which is an X sex chromosome. The second population also has a chromosomal content of 23 but the sex chromosome is Y-shaped and hence called Y.

If the sperm bearing the X chromosome fertilizes the egg, the chromosome complement of the nucleus of the fertilized egg will become 23X + 23X or 46 (XX) and the child will be a girl. If the sperm bearing the Y chromosome fertilizes the egg, the chromosome complement of the nucleus of the fertilized egg will be 23X + 23Y, or 46 (XY), and the child will be a boy (Fig. 5.5).

The fertilized egg now divides to form two cells, then four cells, then eight cells and so on, and each new cell contains the same chromosomal complement, 46XX or 46XY.

In most cultures, each family desires at least one son to carry on the family name, or to see that the spirit of the father goes to the next cycle of existence after death, or to be able to worship his ancestors, or to prove that the man is really a man who can "make many sons."

Because of this desire and because of the patriarchal nature of most societies, many couples would like to be able to choose the sex of their intended child. From time to time reports appear that a doctor, using this or that technique, is able to help couples choose the sex of their child. None of these reports stands up to critical examination. The ancient Greeks thought that men produced boys with sperms from the right testicle and recommended tying off the left testicle to ensure this. The discomfort was great, the results a failure. The method was abandoned.

In more recent times, it has been suggested that the sperms that carry the Y chromosome have a different shape from those that

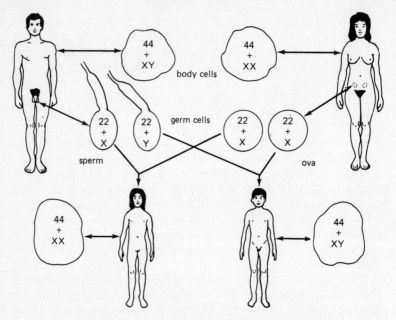

**Figure 5.5** The chromosal determination of sex

carry the X chromosome. The sperms that carry the Y chromosome are claimed to have round heads, those that carry the X chromosome are said to have oval heads. As well as this, the sperm carrying the Y chromosome is claimed to be smaller and lighter than that carrying the X chromosome, and is believed to be more active.

The difference in shape and in weight of the Y-chromosome sperms suggested to Dr. Shettles, who practices in the United States, that because the sperms containing a Y chromosome are different, smaller and more active, they will reach the egg first, if intercourse takes place at the time of ovulation. He has also stated that because the sperm carrying the X chromosome is larger and slower, but stronger, a female child will be conceived if intercourse takes place 2 or 3 days before ovulation and the couple then abstain from sex. Dr. Shettles also believes that the Y-carrying sperm will be helped on its journey if sex takes place at the time of ovulation, if the vagina is alkaline (which means that the woman has to douche before sex), if she has an orgasm either simultaneously with or before the man, if the man inserts his penis in the woman's vagina from behind so that he can penetrate deeply, and if the couple abstain for at least 10 days before having sexual intercourse at the time of ovulation.

In a report of a small series of couples who tried this technique, Dr. Shettles claimed that the desired boy was obtained in a high proportion (85 per cent) of cases.

Unfortunately for this theory, no other investigator has been able to reproduce Dr. Shettles' results. The most accurate investigations have been made when sperms have been put into, and around, the neck of the uterus, using the method of artificial insemination. No preponderance of male children resulted when the insemination was made at the time of ovulation, or of female children when it was done 2 or 3 days before ovulation.

Other researchers have claimed that a preponderance of boys are conceived if intercourse takes place 4 or more days before ovulation. A criticism of the reports of these scientists is that their method of pinpointing ovulation is inaccurate.

Recent research has shown that Dr. Shettles' beliefs are wrong. Scientists have found that if a dye called quinacrine is added to a specimen of semen, about 45 per cent of the sperms show a glowing spot when they are put under fluorescent light. There is some evidence that this glowing spot (sometimes called the "firefly" test) is associated with a Y chromosome, but there is also doubt that the method is sufficiently precise to identify Y chromosomes accurately. Unfortunately, to do the test means killing the sperms, but it has enabled scientists to study the "glow-spot" sperms. The scientists have found that Y sperms do not regularly migrate more rapidly when in an alkaline environment, nor are the glow-spot sperms regularly more active in so far as they migrate further and more quickly. This is the opposite of what Dr. Shettles believes. However, some scientists have found that the male sperms sometimes migrate more quickly in an acid environment. In a series of experiments, Dr. Ericsson found that if he put a natural substance called serum albumin in a long tube, added semen, and then centrifuged the tube, more Y-carrying sperms were found further up the tube. The sperms that had migrated furthest were more uniform in shape that the rest of the sperms, but most of them were exhausted and, when examined, had very poor motility.

In 1979 a group of doctors in Chicago modified Ericsson's method. The technique is complicated. The man masturbates to produce a specimen of semen, which is allowed to become liquid. The semen is then diluted using a special solution (Tyrode's) and is centrifuged for 15 minutes. This forces the spermatozoa to the bottom of the tube. The liquid above the sperms is discarded and the sperms are resuspended in Tyrode's solution. The resuspended sperms are placed at the top of a long glass column, which contains three layers of human serum albumin (HSA). The upper layer consists of the least concentrated HSA. After an hour, the upper layers containing sperms are discarded and after a further half-hour, the lowest layer containing the presumably more active, stronger sperms is collected and centrifuged. This forces the sperms to the bottom of the tube. The liquid on top of them is removed and the sperm pellet is resuspended in Tyrode solution. This is used to inseminate the woman. By 1988 the group and other "franchised" groups reported the results of women treated. The conception rate was low, only 10 per cent of women achieving a pregnancy following a single attempt, and only two-thirds of women sought a second attempt. Following insemination, 457 women became pregnant and gave birth to 336 boys and 121 girls, which means that 74 per cent rather than the expected 51 per cent of the births were of males. It seems that this technique leads to a greater chance of giving birth to a boy, but the birth of a boy cannot be guaranteed.

Other groups are trying to develop techniques to increase the chance of a woman giving birth to a girl, by increasing the numbers of X chromosome (female bearing) sperms, but no reports have been published as yet.

# 6

## Artificial Insemination

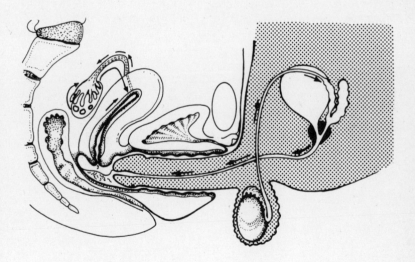

# 6

# Artificial Insemination

In cases where investigations show that the male partner has no sperm in his semen or has a sperm count of less than 5 million per milliliter, pregnancy is either impossible or extremely unlikely. In such cases the only hope that the couple will achieve a pregnancy is by inseminating the woman, at ovulation time, with semen provided by a healthy donor. This is termed AID. Because of the confusion of AID with AIDS, the term donor insemination (DI) is now being used by many people.

In recent years the demand for AID has increased considerably, partly because the procedure is increasingly acceptable to and accepted by the community, and partly because fewer babies are now available for adoption. Women, who previously would have given their baby for adoption, now either have an abortion or give birth and keep the baby. This means that many infertile couples wishing to adopt have to wait for 5 years or longer.

It has been estimated that world wide, over 25 000 babies conceived by AID are born each year. It is accepted that AID is an appropriate procedure that enables about 1 per cent of all married couples to achieve a pregnancy that otherwise would have been impossible (Table 6.1).

## ARTIFICIAL INSEMINATION BY DONOR

The principles involved in artificial insemination by donor (AID) are simple. About ovulation time, as judged by the criteria discussed in Chapter 2, a specimen of semen from a healthy donor, who is unknown to the couple, is introduced into the woman's cervix using a plastic straw attached to a syringe.

**Table 6.1    Reasons for artificial insemination**

|                              | Per cent |
| ---------------------------- | -------- |
| Azoospermia                  | 60       |
| Severe oligospermia          | 30       |
| Zero motility of sperms      | 3        |
| Ejaculatory problems         | 3        |
| Genetically inherited problems | 2      |
| Rhesus incompatibility       | 1        |
| Other                        | 1        |

The practical problems are more complex. First, donors have to be selected and semen has to be obtained. Second, the woman has to be aware of the time of ovulation. Third, the insemination has to take place.

## SELECTION OF DONORS

The donor of semen must be healthy and agree that his semen may be used to impregnate an unknown woman. He has to be screened for physical and mental disease and should have no family history of genetic inheritable disease. It is an added advantage if he is known to be fertile. He is examined physically, and tests are made on his blood to determine his blood and rhesus group, and the absence of syphilis, hepatitis B and C and the HIV virus (AIDS virus). He is also screened for gonorrhea and chlamydial infection. His semen is analyzed to show that his sperms are normal and it is tested for gonorrhea, chlamydia and trichomoniasis (Table 6.2). If he is accepted to be a donor he must agree that he will never make a claim on his biological child, if by any chance he should discover who received his semen.

**Table 6.2    Criteria for selection of donors**

1 Genetic history. Donors screened against a list of congenital and adult conditions

2 Sexually transmissible disease — none must be present

3 Intravenous drug use — donors must not be users

4 If above are negative, the donor has a swab taken from his urethra, which is tested for gonorrhea and chlamydial infections

5 Blood is taken to check for hepatitis B and C, syphilis, human immunodeficiency virus (AIDS virus)

If all the above are negative the donor is accepted

The evalution of the physical and mental characteristics of the donor enables the doctor to make an attempt to match the donor with the husband so that the child may bear some resemblance to him.

The donor's semen can be used in two ways. In the first, the donor masturbates in the clinic or doctor's rooms about 30 minutes before the woman recipient arrives, and then leaves so that the two remain unknown to each other. The woman is inseminated by the introduction of a small amount of the semen into her cervix, by the use of a syringe. The remainder is squirted around her cervix. Some doctors place a cervical cap, which contains the remainder of the sperm, over the woman's cervix. As it is not always easy to predict the time of ovulation with accuracy, the organization required to use 'fresh' semen is complex and time consuming to the woman, the donor and the doctor and because of concern that the donor may have HIV infection, most physicians have now ceased to use fresh semen.

Because of these constraints, most doctors who practice AID obtain semen from the donor at a convenient time and and freeze it. The semen is collected and a small sample checked to exclude infection as mentioned earlier. The remainder of the semen is mixed with a small amount of glycerol, which protects the sperms during the freezing process. The sperm–glycerol mixture is drawn into a number of plastic straws, each of which contains 0.5 milliliters of the mixture. The straws are then cooled and frozen by being placed first in dry ice and then in liquid nitrogen. Secure in the liquid nitrogen container (at $-196°C$), they can remain in suspended animation for several years. It is usual to keep the frozen semen for 6 months so that the donor can be retested for HIV infection 3 months after the donation. When the semen is required for insemination, a straw is removed from the liquid nitrogen container and thawed at room temperature for at least 5 minutes. The straw is then attached to a syringe and the contents are injected gently into the woman's cervical canal.

## SELECTION OF THE RECIPIENT

Most AID services will only accept couples who are in a stable heterosexual marriage, who are over 21 years of age, who are healthy, and who can provide a reasonable standard of care for the child. A few AID services accept single women and homosexual couples.

The woman who is to receive the donated semen must have been investigated to make sure that she is ovulating and that no obstruction exists in her uterus or oviducts that would prevent the donated sperm from reaching the ovum. Her husband (or partner) must be known to have azoospermia or to be severely oligospermic (less than 5 million sperms per milliliter of semen) or to have certain other rare conditions (see Table 6.1). The couple must have been informed about and be aware of the procedure, and are expected to complete a consent form. They must also be aware that pregnancy may not occur in spite of AID over several months, and that there can be no guarantee that the child will have the precise features and coloring of the husband or partner.

These matters are most suitably discussed in a relaxed atmosphere, sometimes with a trained counsellor as well as the doctor, and sufficient time should be made available for questions.

## THE AID PROCEDURE

If AID is to be successful in leading to a pregnancy, the insemination must be made at the time of ovulation. Most clinics prohibit the husband or partner from ejaculating in the woman's vagina in this period lest his semen and the donor's semen interact imunologically thus reducing the chance of conception. Other experts feel that if the husband has sexual intercourse on the day the insemination is performed, he obtains a degree of psychological support, although his rational mind knows that he could not father the child.

The first step is to identify when ovulation occurs. The most widely used method is for the woman to chart her basal body temperature, as discussed on page 30, and to supplement this procedure by checking the mucus secreted by her cervix. At the time of ovulation, the cervical mucus becomes clear, thin and stretchable (when a sample is taken by inserting a finger high into the vagina withdrawing a sample of mucus and then extending the mucus by separating the finger and thumb). If the woman's menstrual cycle is regular, it is relatively easy to identify the period around ovulation, but if the woman has irregular cycles the mucus method is invaluable. The woman's findings of stretchable clear mucus are confirmed at the AID clinic.

In some clinics the level of luteinizing hormone is measured in the woman's urine or the blood each day around the time of ovulation. The woman brings a sample of overnight urine or has a blood sample taken in the morning of the visit. The level of the hormone is measured and 2–4 hours later a result is obtained. A peak LH level, which is two or three times the base level, occurs 12–24 hours before ovulation, and is used to identify when ovulation is expected to occur.

In most clinics the AID procedure is done by a nurse. The woman attends on the day of probable ovulation. She lies on her back and a speculum is introduced into her vagina, which exposes her cervix. The nurse places the straw, which previously has been thawed rapidly and which contains 1 milliliter of semen into the woman's cervix (or occasionally her uterus). The nurse gently expels the semen by attaching the straw to an insemination syringe (Fig. 6.1). The procedure often is repeated daily for 2 or 3 days.

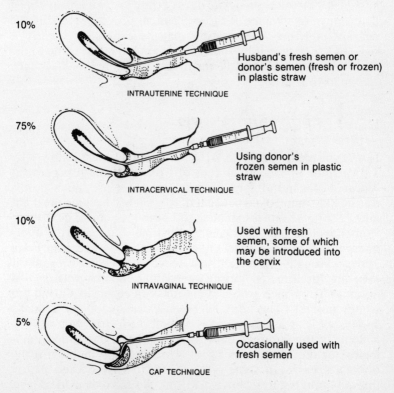

10%

INTRAUTERINE TECHNIQUE

Husband's fresh semen or donor's semen (fresh or frozen) in plastic straw

75%

INTRACERVICAL TECHNIQUE

Using donor's frozen semen in plastic straw

10%

INTRAVAGINAL TECHNIQUE

Used with fresh semen, some of which may be introduced into the cervix

5%

CAP TECHNIQUE

Occasionally used with fresh semen

Figure 6.1  The techniques of AID

Following the injection of the semen the woman usually continues to lie on her back for a short time, makes another appointment and then goes home.

In some clinics the woman is asked to return 5–11 days before her next menstruation is expected, to have the level of progesterone in her blood measured. If the level is below a certain figure, ovulation has failed to occur in that cycle. Between 11 and 20 per cent of women fail to ovulate in the first two cycles of AID. The reason for this phenomenon is unclear, but psychological factors such as anxiety and stress are probably involved.

On an experimental basis, motivated couples who live some distance from the AID center are currently being provided with three straws each containing 2.5 milliliters of semen in a small liquid-nitrogen container, so that the insemination can take place at home. The man is taught how to inseminate his partner and does it on the appropriate days of the cycle, which have been determined in advance. If the experiment proves successful, the concept of home insemination may be expanded. Clearly it reduces the stress felt by some couples in having to come to the hospital; stress may be a factor in the relatively low pregnancy rate following AID.

## HOW EFFECTIVE IS AID?

In any one menstrual cycle, AID at ovulation time is followed by a pregnancy in 10–15 per cent of women. If the procedure is repeated each month for 6 months (unless the pregnancy occurs during this time) 50–60 per cent of women will become pregnant and if the procedure is extended to 12 months, 65–75 per cent of women will become pregnant in this time (Fig. 6.2). It is interesting that some researchers have found that the pregnancy rate varies seasonally; significantly more women become pregnant if they are inseminated during the winter months with semen obtained from men whose donation was collected during the winter months. This may be because the quality of a man's sperms varies seasonally and is highest during the winter.

Some of the failures following AID may be due to immunological factors, the woman's genital secretions immobilizing the donor's sperms. In some AID clinics this is checked before insemination is started, but usually the check is only made after 6 or 12 months of failure.

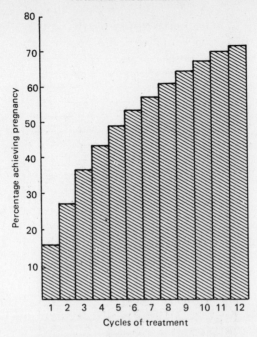

**Figure 6.2** Pregnancy rate after AID

The frequency of miscarriage is no greater after AID than following a natural conception and the progress of the pregnancy is similar.

As mentioned, about 15 per cent of women entering an AID program cease to ovulate for one or several months, perhaps because of stress. Because of this some AID clinics induce ovulation by giving clomiphene from day 5–9, then give an "ovulating" injection of human chorionic gonadotrophin (HCG) on day 13, and perform single intra-uterine insemination about 30 hours later (Fig. 6.3).

# OTHER FACTORS OF IMPORTANCE

## PSYCHOLOGICAL ADJUSTMENT TO AID

Because 25 per cent of women receiving AID fail to become pregnant, and because repeated inseminations may be necessary, some women require psychological help from a counsellor. The opportunity to talk about anxiety and fears helps the woman to adjust to the procedure. Her husband may also need to adjust to

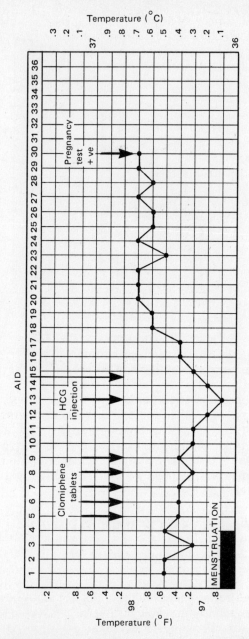

**Figure 6.3** AID following induction of ovulation

the procedure and may ask for counselling. In fact, joint counselling is often helpful and is being requested by increasing numbers of couples. During counselling the man has the opportunity to talk about his anxieties and the possibility that he will be jealous of the unknown fertile donor. He may wish to be reassured about other problems. A positive approach is to compare AID with adoption. A couple adopt a "ready-made child." A couple who choose AID know that half the child's genetic makeup is contributed by his or her mother, and that the husband can experience the pregnancy and, if the couple wish, may jointly experience the birth of their baby.

## HOW STABLE IS A FAMILY AFTER AID?

The evidence shows that the marriage of a couple who have achieved a pregnancy by AID is more stable and long lasting than that of a couple who are fertile. This is probably due to the strong motivation of the couple to have a child and their acceptance of the problems involved. This does not mean to imply that the marriage of some couples who have a child following AID does not break down. Of course, as in the rest of the population, some marriages fail. If a marriage breakdown occurs, the fact that AID was used may be cited as a cause, but in most cases there are other, more significant, reasons for the failure of the marriage.

## HOW MANY OFFSPRING MAY A DONOR PRODUCE?

The reason for limiting the number of donations by a single donor is the chance that two of his progeny might meet, fall in love and have children, who might be genetically abnormal. Most clinics, dealing with a population from a wide area, limit the donations by a single donor to six births to avoid this remote possibility. AID accounts for about one birth in every 1000 live births each year in the community served, so that the chance of a half-brother marrying a half-sister is remote. Even if it occurred, the chance that their baby would be genetically abnormal is less than one in 10. The Warnock Committee in Britain recommended that the number of children born from semen supplied by any one donor be limited to 10.

## UNRESOLVED QUESTIONS ABOUT AID

*Is AID adultery?*

No. In English and Scottish law, adultery presumes some form of sexual intercourse in which the woman's vagina is penetrated by the man's penis. This does not occur in AID.

*Should a child conceived by AID be told of this?*

|  | *For* |  | *Against* |
|---|---|---|---|
| 1 | A person has a right to know his or her genetic origin. | 1 | The biological father can never be found. |
| 2 | The social father or the child's mother avoids committing perjury when registering the birth. | 2 | The child would have to know that his social father was sterile thus impinging on the father's rights. |
|  |  | 3 | The social father is put at a disadvantage, and may be seen as a step-father. |

*Should the donor's semen be mixed with the husband's (or partner's) semen (if any is present), so that the possibility exists that the husband's sperm fertilized the ovum?*

No, mixing of semen reduces the chance of conception, maybe because of possible immunological interaction between the two specimens.

*Are the criteria for selection of AID couples appropriate?*

In some AID services the couple have to pass significant tests before being accepted. These include the following:
1 The woman must be mentally and physically capable of bearing a child.
2 The family environment must be good.
3 The couple should have a reasonable life expectancy.
4 The desire for a child must be that of the couple themselves and not a response to family pressures.
5 The couple must be able to give the child a suitable intellectual chance in life.

The problem in accepting some or all of these criteria is that apart from the first, they are based on subjective value judgements. No such prohibitions are placed on naturally conceived children. It is difficult to know what criteria can be found to quantify such opinions.

One way out of the dilemma of this approach is for the assessor (who is usually a doctor) to be expected to justify his or her opinion why the couple were rejected, rather than attempting to justify why they were selected.

*Are fresh sperms more effective than frozen sperms in achieving a pregnancy?*

In general, the quality and the ability of human sperms to fertilize an egg are reduced if the sperms are frozen and then thawed, probably because of damage to the sperm head during the process. Frozen sperms are probably only 50 per cent as effective in fertilizing the egg in any one AID cycle. Over a 6-months period of AID, 70 per cent of women inseminated with fresh sperms will become pregnant, compared with 35–45 per cent when frozen sperms are used.

*Should AID be restricted to married couples?*

This depends on the philosophy and religious beliefs of the community. The reason for restricting AID to married couples is to "preserve the primacy and integrity of the normal family and to ensure that the child has a stable environment in which to grow." As between 20 and 40 per cent of marriages fail, ending in divorce, separation or constant interpersonal conflict, this reasoning is difficult to sustain. An unmarried couple in what appears to be a stable relationship (whether hetero- or homosexual) can give as much love and care to a child conceived by AID as can a married couple, and the evidence is that such children are as well adjusted, and socially secure as children of married couples.

# THE ETHICS OF AID

Most moral objections to AID have come from the Roman Catholic Church and to a lesser extent from the Lutheran Church and from Orthodox Jews; however, some members of these churches seek AID as a relief of their infertility. This may cause mental conflict because of the condemnation of AID by these churches. The theological reasons for the condemnation is first, that the semen is provided by masturbation, which in the view of the Roman Catholic Church is an "intrinsically and seriously disordered act." Second, the procedure involves a third person in an act that should be exclusively the prerogative of the husband in a marriage relationship. It is held that such an intrusion may debase the marriage, and may lead to undue tensions between husband and wife, although the evidence is that AID enhances rather than diminishes the intimacy of the marriage. Very few couples regret their decision to have AID and most are prepared to recommend the procedure to other couples.

The ethical position of the donor is also in dispute. By donating his semen to an unknown woman, who may then bear his child, he renounces his personal involvement in what should be a significant series of events. On the other hand, the donation may be seen as a compassionate loving gift, which will bring happiness to the couple. In this case the donor has performed a good deed.

A third ethical question involves the child. Has the child the right to know that his or her biological father is an unknown man? Would such knowledge damage the child's psychological development? Is it ethically proper to withhold the identity of the child's biological father from him or her?

The Warnock Committee in Britain has suggested that a child conceived by AID should have the right to know the nature of his or her conception but not the identity of the biological father.

Whatever the ethical problems, a study in 1982 in Scandinavia showed that the majority of parents did not intend to inform their child of his or her true origin, and were most anxious that the details of the insemination were treated with the utmost confidentiality.

These problems should be resolved by a couple seeking AID before the procedure is performed. The evidence is that couples contemplating AID are more concerned about the way they will care for their child and the love that they will give him or her, than couples who give birth following a natural conception.

## AID AND THE LAW

In the past 10 years the use of AID to help women achieve a pregnancy and to give birth has increased dramatically. However, in many countries the legal status of a child conceived by AID is unresolved, and the mother of the child, her husband or partner (unless he is the donor of the sperms) may be at risk of a charge of perjury when completing the birth certificate.

There is a need for precise legislation to answer the questions that may arise from AID. These include the following:
• Is the husband (or partner) of a woman whose child was con-

ceived by AID responsible for the maintenance of that child?

- Is the donor (the biological father) liable for the maintenance of the child, should his identity become known to the mother of the child?
- As the child is not the natural child of the woman's husband (or partner) can he or she inherit any of his estate unless the child is specifically identified as a beneficiary?
- Is a child born by AID, in the absence of legal adoption, the child of the woman's husband (or partner)?
- If the woman, or her husband, completes the Birth Certificate in which the father of the child must be declared (or the space left blank) and declares that he is the father does she or he commit perjury?

These problems could be resolved by legislation similar to that suggested by Justice Asche of the Family Court of Australia:

If a male person consents in writing to be known as the father of a child conceived through artificial insemination and if the woman who is artificially inseminated acknowledges that she accepts such a male person as the father of the said child, such male person shall be deemed for all purposes to be the father of the said child and the said child shall not be the child of the donor of the semen unless he is the person who has signed the said acknowledgement.

Until such legislation is passed, it is prudent for a couple who seek AID and their medical advisers to be aware of existing laws. For example, in England, a child born as the result of AID is illegitimate, the husband's consent to AID being immaterial. The child should be registered as illegitimate, "father unknown" and later (usually 6 months after the birth) he or she should be adopted by the couple.

However, changes may occur. In 1982 a report by a Law Commission on Family Law and Illegitimacy in the United Kingdom, and in 1984 The Warnock Committee on Artificial Reproduction recommended that there be a statutory provision decreeing that the husband of a woman who gives birth to a child conceived following AID be the father of the child, provided he had consented to the AID procedure, and the donor of the semen should have no parental rights or duties relating to the child. This is similar to the suggestion made by Mr. Justice Ashe.

The Warnock Committee further recommended that AID services only be provided on a properly organized basis and be under the control of a licensing authority.

# AID OR ADOPTION?

The alternative to AID is to adopt a baby. This poses several major problems today:

- With the increased availability of abortion, fewer women bear unwanted, unwelcome children, and the number of babies available for adoption has fallen considerably.
- Of those who are unmarried and choose to give birth rather than seek an abortion, over three-quarters now keep their baby.
- In AID in contrast to adoption, both parents experience the pregnancy, participate, if they choose, in the birth and celebrate the birth together.
- If the woman has a desire to bear a child, such a desire cannot be fulfilled by adoption but is fulfilled following AID.
- Following AID, the child has a greater chance of resembling at least one of its parents than an adopted child.
- The legal position of an adopted child is increasingly that when adult he or she has a right to know who the natural mother is, and may wish to see and spend time with her. The knowledge that this may occur may interfere with the relationship between the child and the adopting parents.
- Adoption is only permitted if the adopting parents fulfill certain criteria regarding their age (usually less than 35), financial stability, the marriage relationship and other factors. Much less stringent criteria are used in most AID services.

# ARTIFICIAL INSEMINATION WITH HUSBAND'S SEMEN (AIH)

The ethical and legal dilemma about AID is not applicable to artificial insemination using the husband's semen. If AIH is used there can be no question of adultery. However, the place of AIH in the treatment of infertility is minor and the success rate in terms of a pregnancy is low, fewer than 10 per cent of women achieving a pregnancy following AIH.

The usual method is for 1 milliliter of a fresh semen sample to be injected into the cervical canal at the time the woman is presumed to be ovulating. A few doctors inject the semen into the upper part of the uterine cavity, but research does not show that this results in any increased pregnancy rate. AIH may be appropriate, after the couple have been fully informed, for the few male infertility problems discussed below.

**Oligospermia**  In these cases the number of sperms per milliliter of semen is less than 20 million and the sperm's motility is often impaired. In the only properly designed study reported, the pregnancy rate following AIH in this condition was less than 15 per cent, which is no better than that expected by chance.

As mentioned on page 91, the use of the sperm penetration assay (SPA) may help to identify those oligospermic men whose sperms are likely to fertilize the woman's ovum and those whose sperms are unlikely to do so. If AIH is contemplated it is probable that only the sperms of those men who have a positive SPA test should be used if a higher pregnancy rate is to be obtained.

**Asthenospermia**  In most cases artificial insemination of the husband's asthenic sperm is followed by a very low pregnancy rate. Recent reports record that higher rates have been obtained by selecting sperms that produce a positive sperm penetration assay (see p. 91) and then by processing the semen, so that a more concentrated quantity of motile sperms is obtained. The semen sample is centrifuged in a nutrient fluid and the pellet of sperms at the bottom of the centrifuge tube is removed. It is resuspended in a nutrient fluid, which permits the most active sperms to separate out in a layer at the top of the fluid. This layer, which contains many active sperms, is inseminated into the cavity of the uterus through the same type of narrow plastic tube that is used for embryo replacement.

**Sperm-immobilizing antibodies in the cervix**  Since antisperm antibodies in the cervix (or on the head of the sperm) lead to the failure of the sperms to penetrate the cervical mucus at ovulation time, it is an attractive concept to by-pass the cervix by introducing the sperms into the uterus. Using this technique pregnancy rates of between 10 and 20 per cent have been reported. Once again, similar pregnancy rates occur if no treatment is given, so the value of the procedure is questionable.

**Retrograde ejaculation**  Some men (particularly after a prostate operation) are unable to ejaculate normally and at orgasm ejaculate into their bladder. Urine rapidly damages or kills sperms and little success has been obtained using a procedure in which the man passes urine immediately after orgasm, the sperms are separated by centrifuging the urine, and are then used for AIH. Recently it has been found that if the man overfills his bladder and then reaches orgasm he may ejaculate normally.

**Storage of sperms**  A few men who develop cancers such as leukemia, Hodgkin's disease or testicular cancer may wish to have semen stored in liquid nitrogen for possible future use, as the radiotherapy or chemotherapy needed to treat them may irrevocably damage their sperm-producing capacity. The stored sperm may then be used for AIH.

# 7

# Uterine and Tubal Factors

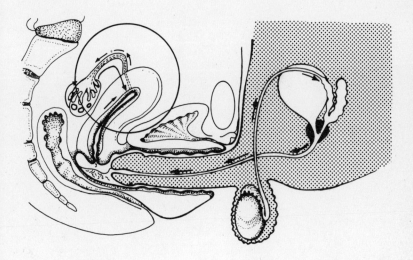

# 7

# Uterine and Tubal Factors

By the time the sperms have penetrated the spiral channels of the cervical mucus and have reached the uterine cavity, their numbers have been reduced considerably. They still have a journey of about 11 centimeters (4¼ ins.) to make before a few will reach the ovum in the oviduct. If the cavity of the uterus is not distorted and if the oviducts are not blocked by infection, the journey of the sperms is relatively easy. However, if the cavity of the uterus is distorted, few sperms will reach the entrance to the tunnel of the oviducts. And if the oviducts are blocked none will reach the ovum. It is also true that if the outer fringe-like ends of the oviducts have been damaged, so that the "fingers" or fimbriae have become stuck together, the ovum, ejected from its follicle, will be less readily picked up, to enter the oviduct. If the fimbriated end of the oviduct has been sealed by infection, the ovum will be unable to enter the oviduct at all. Damage to the inner lining of the oviduct, usually due to low-grade infection, may also prevent pregnancy. Many of the cells lining the oviduct have hairlike fronds or cilia, which beat in unison, forming currents that help the egg to move towards the uterus. If the cilia are damaged, the movement will not occur so readily, and the fertilized egg may linger in the oviduct, where it may cause an ectopic pregnancy. Alternatively it may be moved towards the uterus more slowly than normally and may be unable to settle on to, and implant into, the lining of the uterus.

## UTERINE FACTORS

Uterine causes of infertility are relatively uncommon today. Fifty years ago, about one infertile woman in every 20 had tuberculosis of the uterine lining (endometrium), which altered its nature and made it less able to accept a fertilized egg. Today, in the developed countries of the world, endometrial tuberculosis is encountered very uncommonly. A new advance has made it possible to inspect the interior of the uterus. An instrument, called a hysteroscope, comprising a hollow tube with a series of lenses and a light source, is introduced into the uterus. Some gynecologists routinely inspect the cavity of the uterus when investigating an infertile woman, but most reserve the test for women whose history or whose examination suggests that the lining of the uterus may be abnormal, or its cavity may be distorted by myomata.

Uterine myomata (or fibroids) are non-malignant tumors that develop in the uterus when a number of muscle fibres start growing abnormally. From tiny beginnings they grow slowly to become pea-sized and, as the months or years pass, increase in size to that of a golf ball, a tennis ball or a grapefruit. The fibroid may be solitary or several may grow, enlarging the uterus and distorting its shape (Fig. 7.1). If the fibroids grow outwards, the

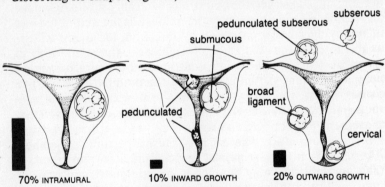

**Figure 7.1**  Fibroids

uterus feels knobbly, whereas if they grow inwards the uterine cavity may be distorted. In this case, the fibroid may hinder the passage upwards of the sperms or may prevent the fertilized ovum from implanting. Should fibroids be found during investigations for infertility, and particularly if they distort the cavity of the uterus, surgery is indicated. The surgeon "shells" the fibroids out of the uterus and reconstructs its shape. Fibroids are not very common in infertile women and are probably the cause of the problem in fewer than one in 300 infertile women.

Another possible uterine cause of infertility is that small adhesions may form in the uterus, usually following a curettage. In severe cases the adhesions cover most of the endometrium, causing amenorrhea and infertility. Whether only a few adhesions have any effect on infertility is unclear, but if found at hysteroscopy, they should be broken.

For many years it was believed that a woman whose uterus was retroverted (tipped back) was infertile. Many operations were devised to correct the abnormal position. It is now known that about 20 per cent of women have a retroverted uterus, that it is not a cause of infertility, and that no treatment is needed, unless there is co-existing pelvic infection.

## TUBAL FACTORS

Damage to the Fallopian tubes (oviducts) usually follows infection of the internal genital organs and is the cause of infertility in about 20 per cent of couples investigated. There is some evidence that an increasing number of young women are developing pelvic infection, or pelvic inflammatory disease (PID), due to chlamydia, gonococci or other sexually transmitted organisms. Pelvic inflammatory disease currently affects about 2 per cent of sexually active women each year. In many cases the infection is symptomless and the woman is unaware she has had pelvic infection. The greater the number of sexual partners the greater is the chance of the woman developing PID. Of the women infected, about one in five will have oviducts damaged to such an extent as to make them involuntarily childless.

An estimate made in the USA suggests that PID results in 200 000 women becoming infertile each year in that country. Whereas increased sexual freedom among women accounts in large part for the increased frequency of pelvic infection, the disease may also follow diagnostic curettage, suction curettage for abortion, or operations such as appendectomy, removal of ovarian cysts or other pelvic operations. After one attack, the proportion rendered infertile averages 14 per cent; after two attacks it rises to 40 per cent and after three attacks to 80 per cent.

Infection may distort the function of the tubes in several ways. It may lead to complete blockage of the tube when the infection damages the interior of the oviduct. Less severe infection may not cause tubal blocks, but may damage the cells that line the interior of the oviduct so that they no longer function properly. Other infections may spare the inner surface of the tubes, but damage the outer surface, so that the oviducts are distorted by adhesions.

Infected oviducts become swollen, and if the swelling is considerable, may be felt when the woman is examined vaginally. But many tubal infections are only discovered when tests are made during investigations for infertility.

## Investigation of the Fallopian tubes

Two methods for investigating the function of the oviducts are currently available. The first, called hysterosalpingography, is to insert a narrow tube into the uterus, through the cervix, and to inject a dye that is opaque to X rays. The second method is to introduce an instrument, called a laparoscope, into the abdominal cavity through a small hole made just below the umbilicus. The uterus and the oviducts are inspected through the laparoscope and a dye is injected through the cervix.

These two procedures have largely replaced an older method of testing the patency of the oviducts. This test, Rubin's test, was developed in 1919 by an American doctor. Dr. Rubin's procedure involved insertion into the cervix of a cannula with a rubber stop on it; the cannula was pressed firmly against the surface of the cervix. Air or $CO_2$ gas was then blown through the cannula and the doctor listened through a stethoscope applied to the woman's abdomen to hear "bubbles." If bubbles were heard, or if the woman complained of shoulder pain when she sat up, the oviducts were declared to be patent. Subsequent development of the Rubin test made it more precise, the pattern of the gas pressure being recorded on an instrument. However, the test only indicated whether at least one oviduct was patent; it gave no information about the condition of the oviducts; false passage of gas occurred; and sometimes gas failed to pass through the oviducts although they were patent. The advantage of the test is that it can be done in the doctor's rooms, but the disadvantages in false results and in the inadequate information the test provides suggest that Rubin's test is now obsolete.

## Hysterosalpingography

This test is performed in much the same way as Rubin's test, in that a tight-fitting cannula is introduced into the woman's cervix (Fig. 7.2). The test is relatively easy to perform but has to be done in an X ray department. If it is performed gently it is not painful, although some discomfort may result.

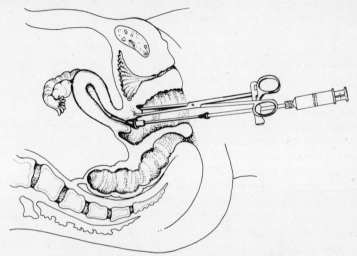

**Figure 7.2**  Hysterosalpingogram—technique

The woman, having passed urine, lies on her back on the X ray table. The doctor examines her vaginally to make sure of the position of her uterus and to confirm that she does not have any evidence of pelvic infection. He cleans her vagina with a mild antiseptic solution and then either introduces a narrow metal tube into her uterus, so that its tip lies just inside its cavity or he attaches a small cap to her cervix by making a vacuum. The metal tube is connected to a syringe, which is filled with a light oily or a water-based substance opaque to X rays. With the use of a television screen the doctor is able to see the tip of the cannula lying inside the uterus as he injects the dye, which fills up the uterus and passes along the oviducts, to drip through their fimbriated ends into the peritoneal cavity. If the oviducts are blocked, the dye will not enter the abdominal cavity. An experienced doctor can derive other information from the pattern made by the dye. The procedure takes about 10 minutes and the woman may be asked to return for a further X ray picture of her abdomen 1 or 24 hours later. At this second visit no instrument is inserted into her vagina.

A normal picture of the uterus (hysteros) and of the oviducts (salpinges) eliminates tubal factors as a reason for the woman's infertility (Figs 7.3a,b). An abnormal picture on the hysterosalpingogram indicates that the test should be repeated or that a laparoscopy should be made (Figs 7.4a,b).

## Laparoscopy

This investigation requires a longer time and is more invasive than hysterosalpingography. Although some gynecologists perform laparoscopy in preference to hysterosalpingography, it is probably preferable to reserve it for cases of abnormal hysterosalpingograms, or if the patient fails to become pregnant within a year of being investigated and found to have no reason for her infertility.

Laparoscopy costs more to perform than hysterosalpingography and is followed by rather more complications, although these are usually minor in nature and affect fewer than 3 per cent of women after laparoscopy.

Laparoscopy is not painless. Following laparoscopy over 50 per cent of women experience pain, of varying severity, for up to 3 days. The pain is usually felt in the upper abdomen or in the shoulder. As well, most women feel that the abdomen is bloated and many experience fatigue, which may last for about a week.

The woman is admitted to hospital for a day and is given a general anesthetic. A narrow needle is inserted into her abdomen, just below the umbilicus, and 2–4 liters of nitrous oxide gas or carbon dioxide gas is injected. This distends the abdomen and pushes the bowel away from its front wall. A small cut is made below the umbilicus and an instrument (the size of a pencil) is pushed into the abdomen. The instrument consists of an outer sleeve (cannula) and an inner solid, sharp-pointed pencil-like instrument (called a trochar). Once the cannula is inside the abdomen the trochar is removed and the laparoscope is inserted through the cannula. The laparoscope is a hollow tube equipped with a system of lenses and a light source. When in position it is possible to inspect the pelvic organs with ease. A cannula, attached to a syringe, has previously been introduced into the uterus, through the cervix, and this is now attached to a syringe

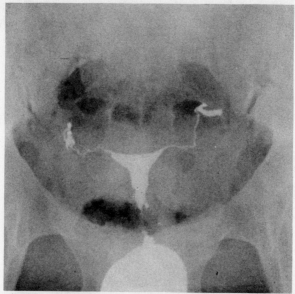

**Figure 7.3(a)**   Patient Fallopian tubes; the dye fills the uterus and outlines the Fallopian tubes

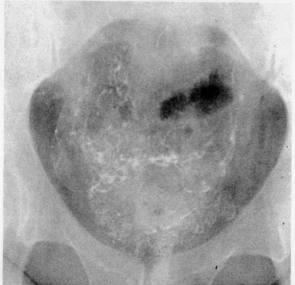

**Figure 7.3(b)**   One hour later — the dye is distributed through the pelvic cavity

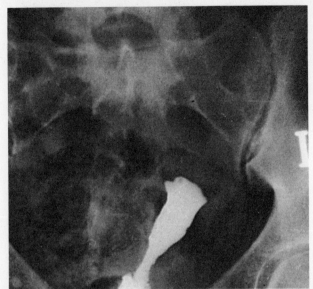

**Figure 7.4(a)**   Blocked Fallopian tubes — the uterus fills with the contrast but none enters the Fallopian tubes

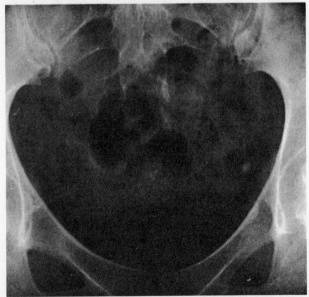

**Figure 7.4(b)**   Blocked Fallopian tubes — no dye is seen in the pelvis in X ray taken 1 hour later

and a dye is injected (exactly in the way that this is done when making a hysterogram).

If the Fallopian tubes are patent the dye will be seen to drip out of the fimbrial ends of the tubes. In addition, adhesions that distort the Fallopian tubes can be seen, and small deposits of endometriosis may be detected. In some women larger patches of endometriosis may be present. These were unsuspected before laparoscopy and unless treated may be a factor in reducing the woman's fecundity. (Endometriosis is discussed on p. 133.)

## TREATMENT OF TUBAL DISEASE

Discovery of tubal disease should be followed by careful evaluation of the damage to the oviducts before strategies for treatment are adopted.

If surgical treatment is contemplated (and this is the usual treatment) the surgery proposed should be explained to the woman and to her partner, and a realistic discussion about the chances of success (in terms of pregnancy) should ensue. The couple need to be aware that surgery is limited to restoring the patency of the oviducts and that it cannot restore their function, particularly the ability of the ciliated lining cells to create movement, if these have been damaged by a previous tubal infection. The surgeon must also make sure that no other major cause of infertility is present (such as male infertility) before carrying out the operation.

Success varies considerably and depends on the degree of tubal damage, the skill of the surgeon in correcting it, and the residual function of the oviducts. Surgery is appropriate in many cases of blockage of the fimbrial ends of the oviducts, provided that the oviduct is not grossly damaged. Surgery is appropriate to cut out a block within the tube (for example after previous tubal ligation) or when the tube is so kinked or distorted that its motility is affected.

Surgery is most successful if the operation is performed by an experienced gynecologist, who performs microsurgery regularly, with the help of some form of magnification. This enables the surgeon to handle the tissues more gently, to use finer instruments and finer sutures, which reduce the reaction of the tissues to the surgical procedure.

Four main surgical procedures are available, depending on the place of damage to the oviduct:

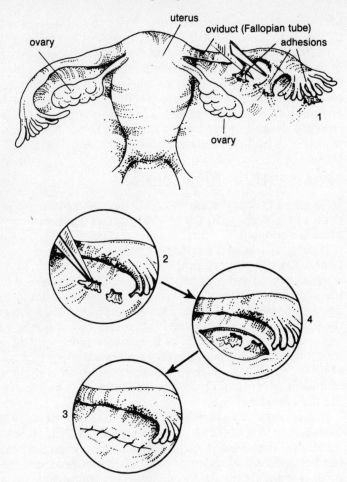

**Figure 7.5**   Dividing adhesions — salpingolysis

- Salpingolysis (fimbriolysis) is the freeing of adhesions that distort or kink the tube (Fig. 7.5).
- Salpingostomy is the creation of a new opening by freeing the fimbria of the tube (Fig. 7.6).
- Tubal anastomosis, in which a blocked section of the oviduct is cut out and the tube reconstructed by joining the undamaged ends (Fig. 7.7). Tubal anastomosis is also used to restore the patency of the oviducts of a woman who has previously had a tubal ligation or sterilization. Such cases, if the damage caused

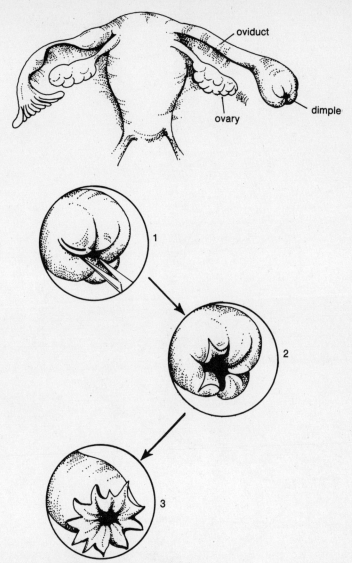

**Figure 7.6** Opening the fimbrial end of the oviduct — fimbriolysis or salpingostomy

by the original operation has not been too great, have the greatest percentage of success, because the function of the tubes has not been impaired, as may occur following pelvic infection.

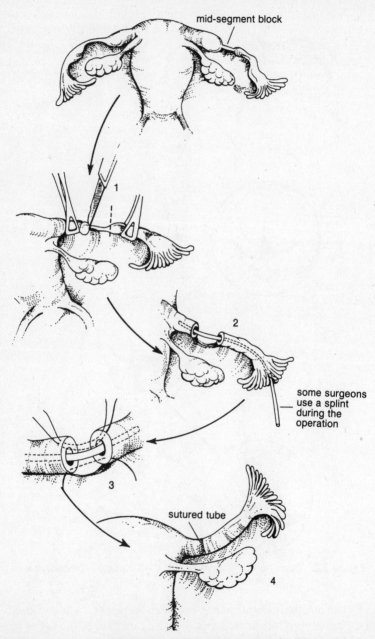

mid-segment block

1

2

some surgeons
use a splint
during the
operation

3

sutured tube

4

**Figure 7.7** Tubal anastomosis

- Tubo-cornual anastomosis or tubal implantation, which is used when the block is in that part of the tube that lies just outside the muscle of the uterus (the cornua). The blocked section of the oviduct is cut out and the patent tube is joined to the patent tube as it emerges from the uterus, or else the tube is implanted into the uterus (Fig 7.8).

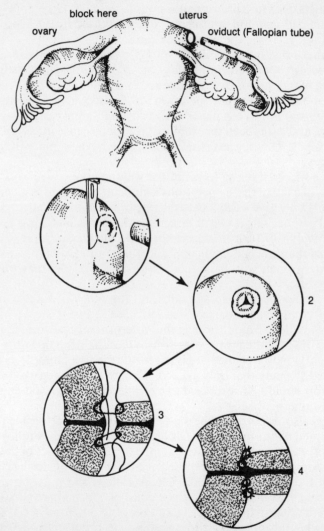

**Figure 7.8** Tubo-cornual anastomosis — microsurgical method

Some surgeons believe that their success rate is improved if the woman is treated by "hydrotubation" at intervals, starting 5 days after the operation. The woman is examined vaginally and a tube is inserted into her uterus. A syringe is attached and a fluid, containing cortisone, is injected so that it passes along her repaired oviducts. The idea is that hydrotubation will help to keep the oviducts open and prevent adhesions forming. It is a painful procedure and a careful multicenter study reported in 1984 shows it does not increase the pregnancy rate.

Other surgeons place plastic splints in the tunnel of the oviduct to keep it open during healing, or in cases of salpingostomy, insert plastic hoods over the opened end. The rod or hood has to be removed by a further operation 5 or 6 weeks later. The value of splints and hoods has never been proven in a properly designed study, and it has been reported that they may cause infection and adhesions. This suggests that, today, they have no place in tubal surgery.

The success rate, in terms of the woman giving birth to a live baby, of each of these operations is difficult to ascertain, as many reports only give a tubal patency rate or a pregnancy rate. As the tubal patency rate is two or three times higher than the pregnancy rate, which in turn is greater than the birth rate because of a higher than normal chance of abortion and ectopic pregnancy among women who have tubal disease, the results may be too optimistic.

In Table 7.1 the average rate, and the range of success rates reported by gynecologists since 1975 are shown.

It is evident from this table that microsurgery performed by a well trained skilled gynecologist provides the woman with a significantly better chance of giving birth to a live child. It can be argued strongly that only gynecologists who have received such training should be permitted to operate on infertile women who have tubal disease.

It is also important that the patient (and her partner) is fully informed about the chance of obtaining tubal patency following surgery. She must also be aware of the increased chance of having an ectopic pregnancy (except in cases of reversal of sterilization, when there is no increased chance). Finally she must be given accurate information about the chance of conceiving and giving birth to a baby. It has to be stated that the outcome in terms of giving birth is not good. Most pregnancies occur in the first year after surgery; a few occur much later.

**Table 7.1 Success rate within 36 months (in terms of the woman giving birth to a live baby), abortion rate and ectopic gestation rate after tubal surgery**

| Operation | Live births | | Result Abortion | Ectopic pregnancy |
|---|---|---|---|---|
| | Mean | Range (%) | (%) | (%) |
| Salpingolysis, fimbriolysis (freeing of adhesions) | 40 | 30–60 | 9 | 4 |
| Salpingostomy: | | | | |
|   Macrosurgery | 15 | 2–20 | 25 | 12 |
|   Microsurgery | 20 | 9–30 | 10 | 7 |
| Tubal anastomosis (after infection) | 20 | 12–40 | 20 | 15 |
| Tubal anastomosis (after reversal of sterilization): | | | | |
|   Macrosurgery | 35 | 10–65 | 15 | 17 |
|   Microsurgery | 60 | 35–75 | 7 | 3 |
| Tubo-cornual anastomosis (or implant into uterus) | 30 | 15–40 | 20 | 10 |

The concern about the relatively poor outcome, particularly in cases of severe tubal damage, led some specialists to suggest that IVF may be the more appropriate treatment. Following IVF (up to three attempts being made) fewer ectopic pregnancies occur, the chance of giving birth to a baby is greater, and the delay in achieving a pregnancy is shorter than after tubal surgery.

# ENDOMETRIOSIS

Endometriosis occurs most frequently in women aged 30–40, and is more common in infertile women. Normally during menstruation the endometrial lining together with tissue fluid and blood is shed through the cervix. In some cases the menstrual discharge passes backwards along the Fallopian tubes, and small fragments of living endometrial tissue fall into the peritoneal cavity, where they may implant on the surface of the ovaries, the oviducts or the uterus (Fig. 7.9). Under certain as yet unknown circumstances the tissue grows, forming a small cyst, which behaves like a miniature uterus. The tissue is acted on by the female sex hormones, and increases in size as menstruation

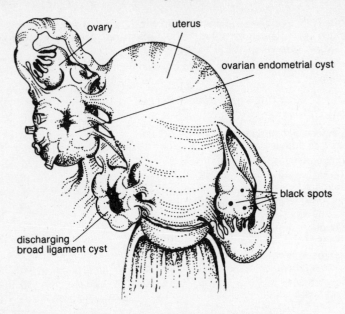

ovary                    uterus

ovarian endometrial cyst

black spots

discharging
broad ligament cyst

**Figure 7.9**  Severe pelvic endometriosis

approaches, shedding its lining tissue at menstruation. But as the blood and shed cells cannot escape, the cyst tends to grow slowly. Most of the blood inside the cyst is absorbed, leaving a tarry black substance. Over the years, the irritation of the tissues surrounding the small cysts leads to scarring, distortion of the tissues and formation of adhesions. Looked at through a laparoscope or at operation, small black lumps, ranging in size from a powder burn or a pinhead to a golf ball, may be seen in the pelvis. Endometriosis may be mild in degree, in which case only tiny areas are seen, usually on the posterior surface of the oviducts or uterus, but there is no scarring, tissue distortion, or adhesions. In more advanced cases, the ovaries have patches of endometriosis on their surface, with scarring, which may also kink or distort the oviducts should any endometrial patches have formed along them. In the most severe cases, the ovaries may be enlarged by endometrial cysts, the size of a golf ball or larger. The oviducts may be involved and there are many adhesions in the pelvis, which may distort and close the oviducts.

It is unclear why women who have endometriosis are more likely to be infertile, except in the severe cases when the damage to the ovaries and oviducts is clearly the factor. In the minor and moderate types of endometriosis, the woman is usually unaware that she has the disease, and it is only detected by laparoscopy. In endometriosis of this degree the Fallopian tubes are not distorted or the distortion is minimal, so that the suggestion that a mechanical action, caused by endometriosis, is the reason for the woman's infertility cannot be sustained.

One rather picturesque theory is that the endometrial tissue produces substances that seduce the ovum away from the entrance to the Fallopian tube. This "Delilah theory" explains little, but it is possible that the endometrial cysts produce prostaglandins that prevent the sperm reaching the egg, or prevent the fertilized egg from being transported efficiently to the uterus. Another theory is that the endometriosis provokes the body to release immunologically competent macrophage cells into the Fallopian tube, where they "eat" the egg or the sperms.

As in much of infertility, controversy continues about the appropriate treatment of endometriosis. If the disease is graded severe, surgery is indicated, either preceded or followed by treatment with a hormone called gonadotrophin releasing hormone analogue (GnRHa) or hormonal drugs called danazol and gestinone. If the disease is graded moderate or mild, most doctors prefer to give one of the hormones rather than to operate.

The drugs act by interfering with the release of gonadotrophins from the pituitary gland, and by reducing the ability of the ovaries to make the sex hormone estrogen. In other words, a "fake menopause" is produced. Ovulation is inhibited, and the endometrium, both inside the uterus and in the endometriotic nodules, is no longer stimulated cyclically. In the uterus, this means that a thin endometrium is produced. This also occurs in the endometrial patches in the pelvis. This permits the fibrous tissue around the endometriosis in the pelvis to invade and to obliterate the small patches, healing them. In a few women the "fake menopause" is accompanied by hot flushes, particularly if GnRHa is used. If danazol or gestinone is chosen, a proportion of the women gain weight, their hair becomes greasy and they develop acne.

Gonadotrophin releasing hormone analogue can be given by injection or the woman may sniff it several times a day. Danazol (and gestinone) is taken by mouth three or four times a day.

Both treatments need to be continued for 6 months. At the end of this time the endometriosis will have disappeared in about

60 per cent of patients, in about 20 per cent only scar tissue will be found, and in the remaining 20 per cent the disease persists.

During treatment the woman is infertile, as ovulation is inhibited. After treatment about 60 per cent of those who had minor disease become pregnant within 2 years (but so do 60 per cent who have no treatment!). About 40 per cent of those women who had moderate disease become pregnant, which is better than if no treatment was given, and about 30 per cent of those who had severe endometriosis become pregnant. Most of the women who become pregnant do so within the first year after the drug treatment is stopped.

These results indicate that the moderate or severe endometriosis found unexpectedly during infertility investigations, and all cases of endometriosis that produce menstrual pain or pain on intercourse, require treatment. The extent and type of treatment depends on the extent of the disease. The more extensive the disease, the greater is the need for surgery, and the lower the subsequent pregnancy rate. Less extensive endometriosis responds to the use of hormonal drugs, especially danazol.

The treatment of minor endometriosis found incidentally during infertility investigations is controversial. Should it be treated or left alone, particularly if it is causing no symptoms and is only found at laparoscopy? If small endometrial cysts are present it is usual to vaporize them with a laser beam or to burn them. Is this enough? The decision is complicated because over two-thirds of infertile women who have mild endometriosis as the only apparent reason for infertility become pregnant within 2 or 3 years of diagnosis without any treatment. The consensus is that drug treatment is of no benefit in mild symptomless endometriosis at least for 18 months.

IVF can be offered to women with endometriosis who have failed to become pregnant naturally. The pregnancy rate in cases of moderate or severe endometriosis is greater if the woman has had 6 months treatment with danazol or GnRHa (as well as surgery in selected cases), but even so the rate is less than if the cause of infertility is tubal damage. It appears to depend on the severity of the endometriosis at the time of diagnosis. If the endometriosis is mild or moderate, between 10 and 12 per cent of women will give birth after IVF (three attempts). If the endometriosis is severe the "take home baby" rate falls to about 5 per cent.

# 8

# Artificial Conception — The New Reproductive Technologies

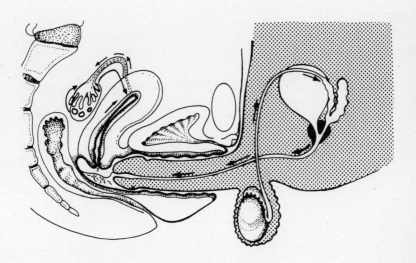

# 8

# Artificial Conception —
# The New Reproductive Technologies

Although "test-tube babies" are a product of the imagination and a fantasy of the "brave new world," in the past decade it has become possible to obtain a woman's ovum, to place it in a test-tube outside her body, to fertilize it with her husband's semen, and when the fertilized egg has divided to become an embryo, to transfer the embryo into her uterus. This is *in-vitro* fertilization and embryo transfer (IVF + ET). In another technique, the egg is obtained and is introduced artificially into the woman's Fallopian tube together with a small amount of treated semen. This is called gamete intra-Fallopian transfer (GIFT). Alternatively the fertilized egg, at an early stage of development is introduced into the Fallopian tube. This is called zygote intra-Fallopian transfer (ZIFT). *In-vitro* fertilization has been in normal use in veterinary practice for many years, but it was not until 1978, when Louisa Brown was born following IVF in England, that the procedure became practical for the treatment of human infertility.

Because the techniques of artificial conception are new, because they deal with a very intimate matter, and because they are concerned with the origins of human life, the ethical and moral aspects of the new reproductive technologies have been, and are, under much scrutiny by scientists, theologians and others. However, there can be no doubt that those couples who achieve a pregnancy by the techniques are delighted.

The techniques are complicated, expensive and time consuming and, for this reason, very careful selection is made, and counselling given before a couple are placed on a waiting list.

# ROLE OF ARTIFICIAL CONCEPTION IN INFERTILITY

The principal reason for offering IVF is that the woman has oviducts that are irreparably damaged following infection, or in whom tubal surgery has failed, as evidenced by the absence of conception in the 2 years after surgery. The clinical observation is confirmed by inspection of the oviducts at laparoscopy and by a hysterosalpingogram. (These rather strict criteria may be made more liberal, in the future, if the success rate for IVF and ET is consistently over 25 per cent, as the pregnancy rate following tubal surgery is lower than this.)

In most services, couples are also included who have unexplained infertility, which is presumed to be due to some undetected problem that prevents the sperm from reaching or uniting with the ovum. The problem may be immunological, anatomical or chemical, but investigations have failed to establish the cause. As pregnancies occur in cases of unexplained infertility to at least 35 per cent of the couples over a period of 5 years of unprotected sexual intercourse, selection of couples on the criterion of unexplained infertility must be strict. At present there is insufficient information to establish appropriate guide-lines.

Some cases of endometriosis are also being treated by IVF or GIFT, which is probably appropriate in cases of severe endometriosis when other treatments have failed to achieve a pregnancy. GIFT is not usually appropriate in cases where the problem is one of tubal damage, but is used occasionally. In some cases of male infertility, IVF or GIFT (and more recently ZIFT) are now being offered as mentioned on page 65.

As more experience is obtained and the results are analysed, the real place of artificial conception will become clearer (Tables 8.1, 8.2).

## SCREENING OF COUPLES ENTERING A PROGRAM

Once couples who might be helped by artifical conception have been identified, further screening is needed before they can be accepted into the program. In most programs, women over the age of 40 are not usually accepted as their fecundity is diminished, although more older women are now being entered into programs. Overweight women are requested to reduce their

**Table 8.1 The place of IVF and GIFT in the treatment of infertility**

IVF is of value in:

- irreparably damaged Fallopian tubes
- unexplained infertility
- sperm antibodies being present in the female genital tract, leading to prolonged (more than 3 years) infertility
- defective sperm function (results generally poor)
- some cases of endometriosis

GIFT (or ZIFT) is of value in:

- unexplained infertility
- ? defective sperm function
- sperm antibodies in the female genital tract
- ? oligospermia

**Table 8.2 Distribution of infertility factors treated by IVF or GIFT***

|  | IVF (%) | GIFT (%) |
|---|---|---|
| Male factors (Ch. 3) | 8 | 12 |
| Tubal problems (Ch. 7) | 47 | 6 |
| Endometriosis (Ch. 7) | 6 | 16 |
| Unexplained infertility (Ch. 10) | 24 | 35 |
| Multiple causes | 2 | 22 |
| Other, not specified | 13 | 9 |

*Series from Australasia and the United Kingdom

weight, as weight reduction increases the chances of conception and benefits the pregnancy. The man's semen is checked, if a semen analysis has not been made recently.

## COUNSELLING

Couples who enter programs for IVF, GIFT, and ZIFT are likely to have considerable stress, anxieties and fears. In most cases the new reproductive technologies are perceived as the last opportunity for the couple to achieve the much desired pregnancy. The couple have been investigated and often treated for many months or years, without success. They may have found it difficult to come to terms with their persisting infertility. The investigations and procedures needed for IVF and the other technologies are invasive, uncomfortable and require the woman to surrender her dignity and her autonomy. This may add to the couple's stress. The knowledge that only one woman in 10 will take home a live and healthy baby after one attempt using IVF, and one in five following GIFT or ZIFT adds to the stress. As well, in most clinics an interval of at least 3 months follows a failure before another attempt is made. During this time the couple may find it difficult to relate, or one or other may become depressed, asking "Why me?"

For these reasons couples embarking on an IVF, GIFT, or ZIFT program need support and counselling. The first and most important way of reducing the stress is for their doctor and the other health professionals with whom they have contact to talk with them, explaining clearly the procedures intended and the probable success rates. The couple should also have the opportunity to ask questions and expect to receive full and honest answers.

The second way of reducing the stress is for the couple to have contact with an informed counsellor who is available to respond to them when problems arise and to diminish their anxieties and fears with minimum delay.

As well as a personal counsellor, many couples find it helpful to join one of the support groups made up of patients and ex-patients so that they can share experiences. This reduces the sense of isolation experienced by some couples. During this time the couple also may wish to consider the ethical implications of artificial conception so that they are certain that they are comfortable about being involved in the procedures.

Artificial conception techniques are complicated and are more easily understood if the process of natural fertilization is first described.

# DEVELOPMENT AND FERTILIZATION OF THE OVUM

By puberty, each ovary contains, randomly scattered through its tissues, about 200 000 tiny primary follicles, the residue of the 2 000 000 that were present during the embryonic period of the individual. Each primary follicle contains an egg (ovum), surrounded by a sphere of several layers of granular cells. Under the influence of the gonadotrophic hormone, FSH, between 11 and 20 follicles are induced to grow each month during the reproductive years. As they grow the cells that surround the ovum first increase in number and, later, secrete fluid that distends the sphere, pushing the ovum to one side, where it lies surrounded by a mound (or cumulus) of cells (Fig. 8.1). The cells of the follicle

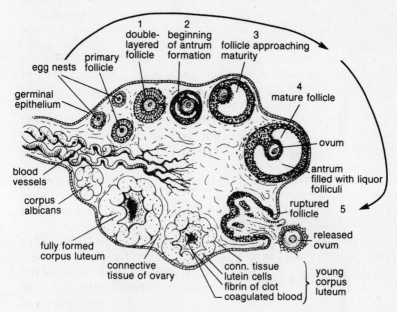

**Figure 8.1** Development of the ovum in the ovary

secrete estrogen, which is taken up into the ovarian veins and from them into the general blood circulation. One of the follicles grows more rapidly than the others and moves through the ovarian tissue to form a bulge on its thickened surface. At midcycle the surge of LH, in some way, induces this follicle to burst, releasing its contained ovum, still inside its cumulus of surrounding cells, and it then enters the fimbriated end of the oviduct.

During the period of growth the ovum has undergone a rearrangement of its chromosomes and has divided equally to form two unequally sized cells, each containing half the normal human complement of 46 chromosomes. The smaller cell resulting from this division is pushed to one side of the sphere (Fig. 8.2).

At the time that the ovum lies inside the oviduct it consists of a nucleus, containing 23 chromosomes, surrounded by a nutritive material, the cytoplasm. The cytoplasm is limited by a surface

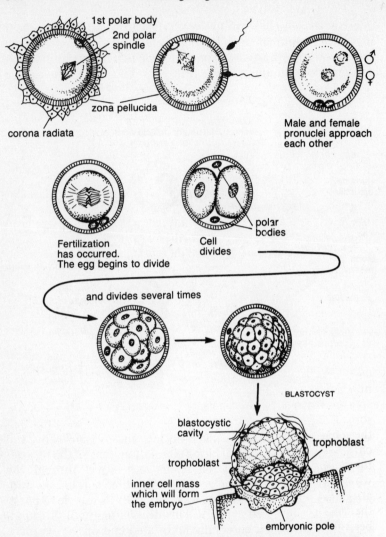

**Figure 8.2** Fertilization, cleavage and development of the ovum

membrane. Outside the membrane is a space, which probably contains fluid, and outside this there is a thickened shell called the zona pellucida. The zona pellucida is surrounded by the cumulus cells, which are adherent to it.

This is how the ovum looks as it is approached by the 30 or 40 sperms remaining from the 300 million ejaculated into the vagina. Of those 300 million, several thousand reach the uterine cavity, and several hundred enter the tunnel of the oviduct; but only a few dozen survive to reach the cumulus cells surrounding the ovum.

One sperm (very rarely two) penetrates between the cumulus cells, and then through the zona pellucida, so that its head lies partly inside the ovum, its tail projecting outwards from the zona pellucida. At this moment, due to the reaction occasioned by the penetration of the sperm, granules of a substance move from the cytoplasm into the space between the surface membrane of the egg and the zona pellucida, preventing any other sperms from penetrating the ovum. Simultaneously the sperm head moves further into the substance of the ovum separating from the tail so that the sperm's head is fully contained in the ovum's cytoplasm. This penetration induces a further significant change in the ovum, which now divides. Each daughter cell has a nucleus containing 23 chromosomes but the cytoplasm divides unequally to form a large cell, the ovum, and a small cell, the polar body, which is pushed by the ovum to the inner surface of the sphere, so that it lies beneath the zona pellucida.

While the cell division is going on, the sperm head embedded in the cytoplasm loses its surface covering, exposing its nucleus. It moves through the cytoplasm to approach the nucleus of the ovum. At this stage the two nuclei are called pronuclei. The pronuclei rapidly fuse to form a single nucleus, a zygote. As the sperm's nucleus (contained in the sperm head) has 23 chromosomes, half the normal human number, when it combines with the nucleus of the ovum, the normal human complement of 46 chromosomes is restored. The advantage of the two divisions of the ovum, which have occurred during its maturation, during which genetic material was exchanged, is that following fertilization, the fertilized ovum has a unique genetic character. With their fusion, and subsequent division, a new biological life has begun.

The fertilized egg divides several times in the oviduct over the next 3–5 days, and during this time loses its attached cumulus of cells, so that its naked, or almost naked zona pellucida marks the boundary inside which the cell divisions take place. After the third division, the fertilized egg consists of identical cells, looking like a mulberry, inside the shell of the zona pellucida. This is the pre-embryo stage. Fluid now seeps between the cells, creating a fluid-filled cavity, with a projecting mound of cells at one side, which will become the embryo, and a layer of cells lining the sphere under the zona pellucida

At this stage the fertilized ovum has reached the uterine cavity. The zona pellucida now becomes fragile and begins to disintegrate, over 2 or 3 days, exposing the sphere of cells, which attaches to and invades the endometrium. Implanting of the fertilized ovum is taking place.

# IN-VITRO FERTILIZATION

The normal fertilization process is mimicked in *in-vitro* fertilization and embryo transfer (ET). The details of the procedure varies between centers, and are constantly undergoing modification to obtain a higher success rate. The following is a typical program.

One month before the date of the *in-vitro* fertilization the couple visit the clinic for a further discussion about the IVF program. The woman is examined vaginally and a catheter, identical in size to the one that will be used to transfer the embryo, is introduced through the cervix. If it does not enter the uterus easily, an anesthetic is given and the cervix is dilated slightly with a small instrument.

There are three stages in the IVF program:
1  Obtaining several fertilizable eggs.
2  Fertilizing the eggs.
3  Replacing the fertilized eggs in the woman's uterus.

## OBTAINING FERTILIZABLE EGGS

In a normal menstrual cycle only one follicle (occasionally two) reaches maturity and releases an egg. In IVF programs there is a need to obtain at least five developed eggs so that the three most healthy and mature can be transferred to the woman's uterus after they have been fertilized.

Several methods of inducing "superovulation" have been devised. Each depends on using hormones to stimulate the development of several follicles. In most programs, clomiphene citrate tablets are taken by mouth in a dose of 100–150 milligrams each from day 2 to day 6 of the woman's menstrual cycle. This is followed by injections of pure follicle-stimulating hormone (FSH) or of human menopausal gonadotrophin (HMG) in a dose of 150 international units from day 5 to day 9 of the menstrual cycle. In some programs, clomiphene is omitted, and HMG or pure FSH is given by injection for 6 to 10 days from the 3rd day of the menstrual cycle, or until at least 3 follicles have reached 18 mm in diameter as measured by transvaginal ultrasound. There does not appear to be any difference in terms of healthy eggs obtained whether HMG or pure FSH is used.

From about the 10th day of the menstrual cycle the growth of the follicles is checked by daily measurements of estradiol in the blood and by ultrasound measurements. In some clinics when the follicles have reached 18 mm in diameter the woman is asked to produce a specimen of urine every 3 hours so that the expected LH rise can be identified (see p. 25). When the rise in LH occurs, or if this measurement is not used, when the level of estrogen in the blood and the size of the follicles are right, another hormone is injected. This hormone is called human chorionic gonadotrophin (HCG). It is obtained from the urine of pregnant women and consists of LH.

HCG induces the final stages of growth of the follicles and maturing of the eggs so that they are ready to be retrieved 34 to 37 hours later.

It should be noted that the technique is still being perfected. For example, some specialists give the HMG injection without monitoring the LH rise. Still other specialists omit giving HCG as they believe that the natural "surge" produces better eggs.

A problem using the clomiphene/HMG method is that in some women the "natural" hormones lead to a spontaneous LH surge before the injection of human chorionic gonadotrophin. This causes the early maturation of some of the eggs. When they are harvested these eggs are not easily fertilized by the sperm.

A way of preventing this is to suppress the release of the gonadotrophic hormones from the woman's pituitary gland. Several methods of doing this are available (see p. 156).

The most successful of them in terms of harvesting healthy, mature eggs, obtaining a higher rate of implantation and a higher "take home healthy baby" rate appears to be the use of a gonadotrophin releasing hormone analogue (GnRHa) which is started on the first or second day of the menstrual period. GnRHa may be given by injection under the skin or by nasal sniffs. On the third day, HMG injections are started and the GnRHa is continued until the follicles are 18 mm in diameter. The rest of the technique is that described earlier.

Early results of this new technique show that the pregnancy rate and the "take home healthy baby" rate is nearly twice as high

compared with when clomiphene is used. However the cost of the
hormones used is much greater.

Women choosing these techniques for obtaining several eggs
should also know that in about 5 per cent of women treated, the
hormones used to produce "superovulation" may cause the
ovaries to become very large. The woman develops abdominal
pain, fluid in her abdomen, a fall in blood pressure and in one-
third of cases life threatening blood coagulation changes. The
condition is called the "ovarian hyperstimulation syndrome." In
time the ovaries usually get smaller, but some women become
seriously ill and a few require operation.

Specialists try to avoid this happening by the most meticulous
monitoring using the measurements of estrogen in the blood and
ultrasound, but in spite of this, ovarian hyperstimulation may
occur. If the blood level of estrogen is exceptionally high, the
attempted IVF is abandoned and the injection of HCG is not
given.

## Preparation of the couple for egg retrieval

Between day 7 and day 9 of the stimulated cycle the couple visit
the clinic to discuss the program and to have their questions
answered. A vaginal swab is taken from the woman to make sure
that she has no vaginal or cervical infection. The couple are asked
to avoid sexual intercourse until after the eggs have been replaced
in the woman's uterus.

Some cycles have to be cancelled because the eggs have developed too rapidly or have failed to develop satisfactorily as judged
by the LH levels in the woman's blood and the ultrasound examinations. Provided the eggs have developed normally, egg pick-
up is scheduled.

## Retrieving fertilizable eggs

Two methods of retrieving the eggs from the ovaries have been
developed. The first is by needle puncture and the second is by
laparoscopy.

**Needle puncture** The development of a vaginal ultrasound
probe has enabled specialists to visualize the ovaries clearly and
to obtain the eggs. A special needle is passed along the probe
under ultrasonic guidance and is pushed forward until its tip is
inside one of the stimulated follicles. By using gentle suction, the
contents of the follicle are sucked through the needle into a test
tube. The needle is then advanced to penetrate the next follicle,
and the egg is sucked out. In this way several eggs are obtained

(Fig. 8.3). The procedure is made under local anesthetic and the woman watches it on the ultrasound screen as it happens. She does not need to be admitted to hospital.

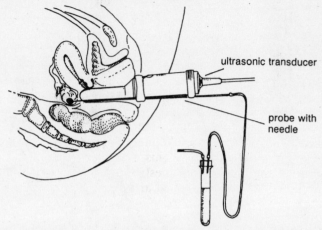

ultrasonic transducer

probe with needle

**Figure 8.3**   Egg pickup using ultrasound-directed needle aspiration

This new technique is much less invasive and painful than laparoscopic egg pick-up. It means that women may feel inclined to have several attempts at IVF, which increases their chance of becoming pregnant and taking home a baby. At present, using the laparoscopic technique, about 20 per cent of women drop out of the program after one attempt.

**Laparoscopic retrieval**   In this technique the woman has to be admitted to hospital and is given a general anesthetic. The laparoscope is introduced into the abdomen through a small incision just below the umbilicus and the ovary is visualized. A long needle is thrust into the abdomen and its point advanced until it enters a follicle. The contents of the follicle are sucked into a test tube. The procedure is repeated until several follicles have been emptied (Fig. 8.4).

After this procedure has been completed the woman may go home and will be asked to return 3 days later for embryo transfer, provided healthy embryos have developed.

## FERTILIZING THE EGGS

### Preparation of the harvested eggs for fertilization

The material sucked out of each follicle is transferred to a test tube or a flat glass dish. The "egg scientist" examines the material

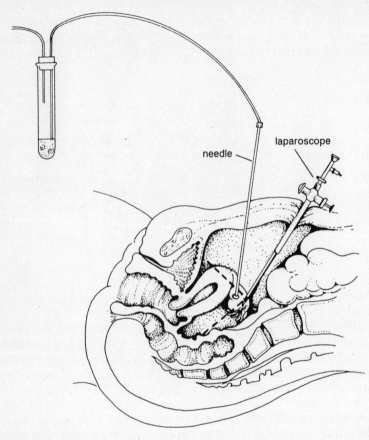

Laparoscopy is performed 26–28 hours after the LH rise or 36 hours after HCG injection

**Figure 8.4**  Laparoscopic egg pick-up

through a dissecting microscope and teases out the eggs so that they are free from blood. They are transferred into a test tube containing a culture medium and are incubated for 3–12 hours and then re-examined (Fig. 8.5). The healthy "good" eggs are selected for fertilization.

## Preparation of the semen

The woman's husband, meanwhile, has produced a specimen of his semen by masturbating in the laboratory. The specimen is

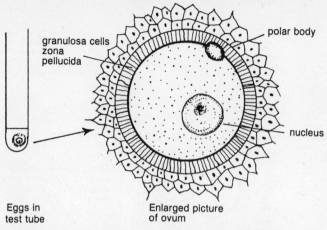

granulosa cells
zona
pellucida

polar body

nucleus

Eggs in
test tube

Enlarged picture
of ovum

**Figure 8.5**  Preparation of the eggs for fertilization

centrifuged and the sperms are washed once or twice in a special
fluid. They are then placed in a test tube containing a culture
medium for about 2 hours. In one Swedish IVF center an inert
substance, obtained from connective tissue, is mixed with the
culture medium, which increases its viscosity. The Swedish
scientists believe if they do this only the best, most active, sperms
will swim to the top layer of the culture medium. These select
sperms are used to fertilize the eggs.

When the incubation period is completed, the specimen is
examined under a microscope, and a sample containing about
50 000 sperms is added to each of the culture tubes, which contains an egg. In a few IVF clinics the remainder of the sperms are
injected into the woman's vagina. The scientists who do this
believe that it results in a higher pregnancy rate, and they
speculate that the sperms swim up into the uterine cavity and, in
some way, excite a response from the endometrium, which
makes it more receptive to the implanting embryo.

The sequence of illustrations in Figure 8.6 shows what happens
in *in-vitro* fertilization.

## EMBRYO TRANSFER

The fertilized eggs are checked by being scanned with a stereo
microscope about 18 hours after insemination. Unfertilized eggs
or abnormal-looking eggs are discarded. Another scan is made

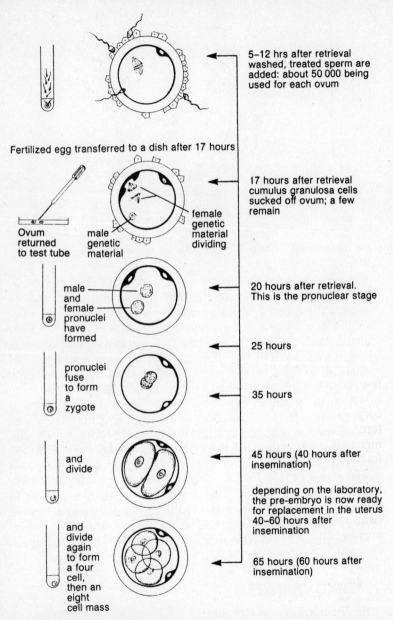

5–12 hrs after retrieval washed, treated sperm are added: about 50 000 being used for each ovum

Fertilized egg transferred to a dish after 17 hours

17 hours after retrieval cumulus granulosa cells sucked off ovum; a few remain

female genetic material dividing

Ovum returned to test tube

male genetic material

male and female pronuclei have formed

20 hours after retrieval. This is the pronuclear stage

25 hours

pronuclei fuse to form a zygote

35 hours

and divide

45 hours (40 hours after insemination)

depending on the laboratory, the pre-embryo is now ready for replacement in the uterus 40–60 hours after insemination

and divide again to form a four cell, then an eight cell mass

65 hours (60 hours after insemination)

It is now ready for embryo transfer

**Figure 8.6** In-vitro fertilization of the eggs

about 50 hours after insemination, when the fertilized eggs are at the four-or eight-cell stage, to make sure that they are healthy and developing normally. It is important that these checks are made because only about 40 per cent of the eggs will be fertilized and develop normally. Some of the healthy eggs are chosen to be replaced in the uterus, when it is hoped that they will implant into its lining.

Another method to determine if the fertilized eggs (embryos) are healthy has been developed in Sydney, Australia. In this, a small amount of the culture fluid is injected into mice that have had their spleens removed. If the embryo is of good quality, the injection leads to a fall of 20–40 per cent in the mouse's blood platelets. This is thought to be due to a substance produced by healthy embryos. The group claims that more eggs are fertilized and develop into healthy embryos if this substance, which has been called the "platelet activating factor," is added to the culture medium in which the fertilized eggs are grown.

Provided two or three good eggs are obtained, the woman is contacted and she returns to the clinic or hospital for the transfer. This is done by sucking the fertilized eggs gently into a very narrow catheter, which is then gently introduced into the woman's uterus through her vagina. The eggs are then gently transferred into the uterine cavity (Fig. 8.7).

After the embryos have been transferred the woman rests for a few hours in the clinic or the hospital. Some specialists give an injection of HCG 2 and 4 days after the transfer to encourage the corpus luteum (see p. 25) to produce a greater amount of progesterone. This is thought to improve the quality of the endometrium, making it a more "fertile soil" in which the embryo finds it easier to implant.

There is some controversy about how many of the fertilized eggs (embryos) should be transferred. If too many embryos are replaced in the uterus a high rate of multiple pregnancies (usually twins) may be expected. If too few embryos are transferred none may implant. Current opinion suggests that the transfer of three embryos is the optimal number, but recent reports from London indicate that transferring two healthy embryos gives better results in terms of healthy "take home" babies and a reduction in the number of multiple pregnancies.

Pregnancy can be diagnosed 9–14 days after the transfer by measuring the pregnancy hormone, β-HCG, in the woman's blood. Some scientists measure β-HCG on days 9, 17 and 25 to

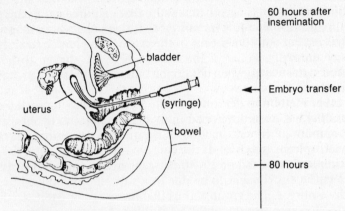

60 hours after insemination

Embryo transfer

80 hours

A special catheter made of Teflon (called a "Tom Cat") introduced into the uterus; two or three embryos, with a small amount of culture medium, are injected into the uterus.

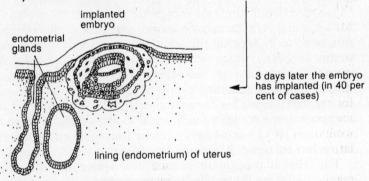

3 days later the embryo has implanted (in 40 per cent of cases)

**Figure 8.7** Embryo transfer to the uterus

help them decide if the pregnancy is going to continue. A low HCG on day 9 and day 14 suggests that the embryo is dying. A low HCG on days 17 and 25 indicates that the pregnancy has failed as the embryo is "blighted" and is dead. It is usually absorbed by the woman's body but in a few cases she will have the symptoms of a miscarriage.

Between 35 and 45 per cent of the transferred embryos implant. Half of them produce a "biochemical pregnancy" (HCG is detected in the blood) and then die. Between 55 and 65 per cent survive but about one-quarter of them miscarry and a few develop in the Fallopian tube, forming an ectopic pregnancy. This means that if the woman reaches the embryo-transfer stage, she has a 15–20 per cent chance of delivering and taking home a healthy baby. As has been explained, not all women entering an IVF program reach the state of having an egg retrieval. Of those who do, in only four out of five women are four or more healthy eggs obtained.

These data mean that a woman who enters an IVF program has a 10–14 per cent chance of giving birth to a healthy baby. If she has several attempts, the statistical chance of having a "take home" baby increases; if she has four attempts she has about one chance in five of conceiving and giving birth to a healthy mature baby. However, practical experience, reported from the USA, indicates that 8 out of every 10 births occur to women in the first two treatment cycles.

# REFINEMENTS IN IVF AND GIFT

## IVF FOLLOWING NATURAL OVULATION

Most clinics performing IVF found that they obtain a higher pregnancy and "take home" baby rate if they induce the woman to superovulate as described on page 146–7. However, inducing a woman to superovulate is expensive because of the cost of the drugs, the laboratory tests required and the time involved, both for the woman and for the staff of the clinic. This has led to a reappraisal of the original approach to IVF, namely to let the woman ovulate spontaneously, and retrieve the egg when ovulation has occurred.

The technique can only be used if a woman has reasonably regular ovulatory cycles. Her menstrual cycle is checked for 3–6 months to determine its regularity. Once this has been determined the woman is given an injection of human gonadotrophic hormone 2 days before the anticipated day of ovulation. A single egg is obtained using the transvaginal probe under local anaesthesia. The woman brings a fresh sample of her husband's semen when she attends the clinic for egg retrieval. If the egg is fertilized she returns for the embryo implantation 2 days later. The chance of achieving a 'take home' baby after one attempt is about 7 per cent, but as the procedure only takes about 30 minutes for each of the two visits, it can be repeated more often than IVF following superovulation. The cost is about one-quarter that of IVF following superovulation and, as has been mentioned, permits a saving of time for the IVF center staff and for the woman herself.

## HORMONE MANIPULATION

As mentioned earlier several techniques are being tried which suppress the woman's pituitary gland function and so stop the release of her own FSH and particularly, LH. This prevents an early surge of LH which is the cause of the problem of poor fertilization of the eggs.

In the first method the woman takes the Pill during the menstrual cycle preceding the IVF attempt. On the third day after stopping the Pill, either clomiphene and HMG are given or HMG alone is given, as in the usual method of stimulating the ovaries to superovulate to obtain eggs for IVF (see page 146). Another method is to give the woman tablets of the synthetic hormone progestin from the middle of the cycle which precedes the IVF attempt. Between 3 and 5 days after the hormone treatment is stopped the woman has a "withdrawal bleed." On the second day of the bleed, she is given clomiphene and HMG as described earlier and the "egg pick-up" is fixed for day 13 or 14. These methods seem to have had no benefit over the older techniques.

The failure of these techniques to produce a higher pregnancy and "take home" baby rate has led to the development of the use of a laboratory made hormone called gonadotrophin releasing hormone analogue (GnRHa), in a dose higher than that usually released by the pituitary gland. This has the paradoxical effect of suppressing the release of the woman's own gonadotrophic hormones (FSH and LH). She sniffs GnRHa five times a day, or is given injections of the hormone, either from day 21 of the menstrual cycle preceding the one in which the attempted IVF will be made, or from the first day of the period during which IVF will be attempted. In the first case, 18 days after starting the GnRHa, HMG is started, and she receives both hormones. This method is described on page 147.

## DONOR OVA

Women whose ovaries have been removed by surgery, or who have ovaries that do not contain any ova, as in Turner's syndrome, can now be helped to have a baby. So can women who have premature ovarian failure (premature menopause) and women who carry a gene for a genetic disorder. The technique is to use a donor's eggs. Ethically this technique is no different from a semen donation needed for AID.

The woman's uterus is prepared for pregnancy by giving her sex hormones to mimic the hormones secreted in a normal menstrual cycle. On the 16th, 17th or 18th day of the "artificial" cycle, which may be manipulated to coincide with the same day of the donor's cycle, eggs are obtained from a donor, and these are fertilized *in vitro* by the woman's husband's sperms. The resulting embryo is placed in her uterus using the technique of the IVF program.

The eggs may be donated by a woman undergoing IVF on the same day; by obtaining eggs from a volunteer donor who is having a tubal ligation performed on the same day, by a relative or by using frozen eggs. In the future it may be possible to obtain eggs from their unstimulated follicles in the ovaries and treat them so that they develop in a test tube as they would in the ovary during the menstrual cycle.

# EMBRYO TRANSPLANTATION

In this technique a "donor mother" agrees to be inseminated by the sperm of the husband of the infertile woman. The infertile woman's menstrual cycle has been synchronized with that of the donor mother by the use of hormones. The insemination is made at the time that the "donor mother" ovulates. If a pregnancy results the embryo is "washed out" of the donor mother's uterus a few days after fertilization, before it has implanted and is transplanted into the infertile woman's uterus.

The ethical problems associated with this technique are considered on page 171.

# THE USE OF FROZEN EMBRYOS

Recent research has shown that if an embryo at the four- or eight-cell stage (it is often called a pre-embryo at this stage) is frozen in liquid nitrogen, it may be replaced in the mother's uterus at a later date with the same or a greater expected chance of developing into a healthy baby, as with the transfer of a fresh embryo. The development of the technique has spared some women from having repeated laparoscopies, or vaginal retrievals to collect eggs, should the first attempt at IVF and ET fail.

The patient is induced to superovulate and between six and twelve eggs are obtained. The eggs are checked and healthy eggs are fertilized *in vitro*. Two or three pre-embryos are transferred to the mother's uterus and the remainder are frozen in liquid nitrogen. If the transferred eggs fail to produce a "take home" baby, a second attempt is made using two or three of the frozen pre-embryos.

The advantage of this technique is that the woman does not need to undergo a second laparoscopic or vaginal egg retrieval should the first attempt fail.

Of course, the procedure has to be controlled by strict ethical rules. A further ethical problem arises if the woman becomes pregnant and delivers a live baby at the first IVF attempt. What should be done with the frozen pre-embryos? This problem is discussed on page 168.

# THE SUCCESS RATE OF IVF

Reports from various IVF clinics use different criteria to determine their success rates. Some report numbers of pregnancies achieved per laparoscopy performed; others report pregnancies per embryos transferred; others report pregnancies per woman entering the program.

For the infertile couple the only successful outcome is a healthy "take home" baby.

What are the chances of this being achieved?

If the results of the most efficient, well-conducted clinics are analyzed some answers can be obtained. Of 100 women entering the IVF program, 10 will either drop out or become pregnant before the first IVF attempt. Ninety women will be prepared by taking hormones to superovulate so that a transvaginal or laparoscopic egg collection can be made, and in 85 women eggs will be harvested. The eggs are fertilized in a test tube and the early embryos are examined through a stereomicroscope. In 80 women, at least one, and preferably, three "good" embryos are found and are transferred into the woman's uterus. About one-quarter of the embryos manage to implant, so that 20 women will become pregnant. About one-third of the pregnancies will fail to reach the 20th week of pregnancy because the apparently healthy embryo either dies very early (a biochemical pregnancy) and this happens to about 5 per cent of the implanted embryos, or dies a bit later (a blighted embryo — about 18 per cent of the implanted embryos) or miscarries (6 per cent) or implants into a Fallopian tube causing an ectopic pregnancy (5 per cent).

This means that a single attempt at IVF will be followed by a "take home" baby in between 9 and 14 per cent of women, but one-third of the babies will be premature, weighing less than 2500 grams at birth. Most of these premature babies are one or both of twin or triplet births and unfortunately some of them die. Twin births (and occasionally triplet births) are much more common after an assisted conception (20 per cent) than after a natural conception (1 per cent). Three per cent of births are of triplets. As much as the couple have desired a pregnancy, a twin birth and particularly a triplet birth may cause considerable emotional and financial stress on the couple. The stress is diminished if the couple have had the opportunity to explore their feelings should a multiple birth result from the artificial conception program. (Table 8.3).

**Table 8.3   The chance of giving birth to one or more babies following one IVF attempt\***

|                                                                 | Number | %    |
| --------------------------------------------------------------- | ------ | ---- |
| Accepted into program                                           | 1000   | 100  |
| Laparoscopy performed                                           | 850    | 85   |
| Ova obtained                                                    | 800    | 80   |
| Ova fertilized                                                  | 700    | 70   |
| Embryos (2 or 3) transferred                                    | 600    | 60   |
| Clinically pregnant                                             | 180    | 18   |
| Abortion or ectopic pregnancy occurs (33%): Remaining pregnancies | 120    | 12.5 |
| Live birth ("take home" baby—30% are premature)                 | 112    | 11.2 |

\*Based on information reported to the National Registries in Australia and the United States of America, 1987–1990.

# OTHER METHODS OF ARTIFICIAL CONCEPTION

## GIFT

GIFT (gamete intra-Fallopian transfer) has been developed to overcome some of the problems of IVF, and may achieve a higher pregnancy rate. GIFT can only be used if the woman has at least one patent Fallopian tube. At present, the technique is being used for a variety of infertility problems (see Table 8.2, p. 141). The

woman is superovulated and ova are obtained using IVF
techniques. The three or four best ova are selected. The man
produces a specimen of his sperms by masturbating. The sperms
are treated and 10 000–100 000 of them are taken in a measured
sample and divided into two equal portions. One portion is fed
into a narrow tube (catheter), and then two or three eggs are
drawn up, separated from the semen by a tiny bubble of air. The
second portion of the semen is drawn into the catheter, again
separated from the eggs by an air space. Under laparoscopic
vision the catheter is introduced into the woman's Fallopian tube
and the contents expelled. The procedure may be repeated on the
other Fallopian tube although it is uncertain if this increases the
pregnancy or "take home" baby rate.

The technique permits fertilization to occur in the natural
environment of the Fallopian tube, which should improve the
pregnancy rate.

GIFT is associated with a "take home" baby rate of about
20 per cent, which is higher than that obtained by IVF.

## ZIFT

The technique of ZIFT (zygote intra-Fallopian transfer) also
known as PROST (pronuclear intra-Fallopian transfer) is similar
to that of GIFT. The ova are fertilized by sperm using the IVF
technique. Three of the resulting fertilized eggs, at an early pronuclear stage, when the zygote has just formed, are transferred
into the fimbrial end of the Fallopian tubes as in the GIFT
technique. Whether ZIFT will produce more "take home" babies
than GIFT is not yet known.

# PRECONCEPTIONAL ADOPTION

In this procedure a fertile woman makes a contract with a couple
in which the wife is infertile. The contract stipulates that the male
member of the infertile couple either has sexual intercourse with
the fertile woman at the time she ovulates or arranges for the
artificial insemination of his semen. If pregnancy results, the fertile woman, now a surrogate mother, agrees that following childbirth, the child will be given to the infertile couple. The legal and
moral problems associated with IVF surrogate motherhood
(p. 172) apply in preconceptional adoption. Whatever the legal
and moral problems, it is likely that preconceptional adoption is
being used by certain infertile couples.

# THE PLACE OF ARTIFICIAL CONCEPTION IN THE MANAGEMENT OF INFERTILITY

IVF, GIFT, and similar techniques are being undertaken in about 15 countries, by over 200 teams, and the numbers are increasing each year.

The drug regimens used to induce the woman to superovulate differ between the teams, as mentioned on pages 146, 156, but when the results are analyzed it does not seem to make much difference which regimen is used. A few teams let the woman ovulate spontaneously but fewer pregnancies result, as most women produce only one egg each month and it has been shown that if three or four embryos are transferred to the uterus, the pregnancy rate is higher.

The new reproductive technologies are complicated, time consuming and require the skills of an experienced team of physicians, biological scientists, technicians and counsellors to ensure that the best results are obtained, both physically and psychologically.

Research continues to improve the results and to reduce the emotional and financial costs to the couple.

# 9

## Ethics of the
## New Reproductive
## Technologies

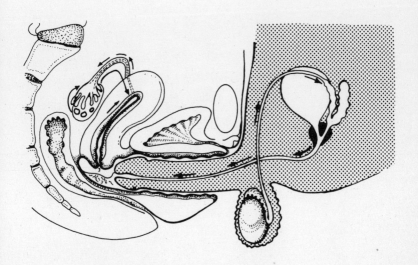

# Ethics of the New Reproductive Technologies

In 1968, the United Nations Conference on Human Rights held in Teheran, reaffirmed that basic right of all couples to have the freedom "to decide responsibly the number and spacing of their children, and for the rights of children to be wanted and cared for." The Declaration then stated that "in order to exercise these rights people must have access to information, education and services appropriate to their needs." Although this Declaration applied to fertility control it is equally applicable to fertility enhancement, including methods of artificial conception.

The considerable ethical problems raised by IVF, following its introduction into clinical medicine, led to the establishment of committees of inquiry in Australia, Britain and the USA. These committees had reported by 1984 and their recommendations were remarkably similar. The committees agreed that artificial conception programs should be controlled by a National Licensing Authority, or, in the case of the USA, by Institutional Review Committees. The Authority or Review Committee would license and inspect clinics where the new reproductive technology was practiced, and would regulate research. This is an important step in defusing the concern about artificial conception, but many people sincerely believe that artificial conception is ethically and morally wrong.

The ethical and moral considerations are discussed in this chapter, under several headings:
• Ethical and moral implications of artificial conception.
• The use of embryos for infertility research.
• Embryo transplantation.
• Surrogate motherhood.
• Who should obtain the new reproductive technologies?

# ETHICAL AND MORAL IMPLICATIONS OF ARTIFICIAL CONCEPTION

The arguments presented below are those of people who oppose the new reproductive technologies on ethical or moral grounds and those who believe that they are ethically and morally beneficial to infertile couples.

*Artificial conception leads to the destruction of "the unitive and procreative aspects of marriage," the destruction of the conjugal act and the removal of natural bodily love between two married persons. Artificial conception, therefore, is dehumanizing, degrades the sanctity of marriage and weakens the family.*

Sexual intercourse, with intravaginal ejaculation of semen, may be an act of love and may sanctify marriage, but it may be forced by a demanding husband on an unwilling wife. It does not guarantee a happy family relationship. Couples who choose to have artificial conception to achieve a wanted pregnancy have been investigated extensively and may have waited for months to have the procedure performed. They are responsible people in a stable relationship. The evidence is that following the procedure the love between the couple is increased not diminished.

*The new reproductive technologies are unethical because the medical scientists are manipulating nature.*

Any medical treatment manipulates nature. Nature, left alone, would ensure that women received no pain relief during childbirth; that the risks to the fetus in pregnancy, which could lead to its death in the uterus, were not recognized or treated; and that infertility problems were not investigated.

*The new reproductive technologies lead to a high loss of human embryos.*

The problem is, first, one of definition. When does a fertilized egg become an embryo? This is important, as the two entities are confused in many people's minds. Following fertilization a delay of about 12 hours occurs before the fertilized egg divides to form two identical cells. Subsequent divisions occur over several days until a bunch of cells is formed, in which a fluid-filled cavity appears (the blastocyst). This is the pre-embryo stage. Most of the cells of the blastocyst will form the placenta, a few cells on the inner surface of the blastocyst will form the embryo. Thus the embryo is formed between 7 and 12 days after fertilization. In current artificial reproduction programs, fewer than one fertilized egg in four is available for implantation, most being lost before the embryo is formed.

Research on fertilized eggs is needed to increase the number of healthy embryos that will implant and will develop into healthy babies. Surely, there can be no objection to carrying out such research before the embryo has formed, as at this stage of its development it has no "personhood." It would also be noted that probably about half of the eggs fertilized following sexual intercourse fail to develop to the embryo stage.

If the embryo stage is reached, the loss following artificial conception is about twice the loss that follows a natural conception.

*There is some reason to believe that artificial conception leads to defective offspring.*

This is false. A child conceived by artificial conception has the same chance of developing normally in the uterus and after birth as a child conceived by sexual intercourse. The proportion of congenital abnormalities among children conceived by IVF or GIFT is no greater than that among children conceived "naturally." Children artificially conceived have no greater risk of mental or physical abnormalities, although more are born weighing less than 2500 grams (5½ lbs.).

*If a child born following IVF or GIFT has a congenital defect or develops a health problem, the parents may feel guilty or suspicious that the new reproductive technology used was the cause of their child's abnormality.*

Most parents feel unhappy and some feel guilty if their child is born with a congenital defect. There is no evidence that parents of a congenitally defective child born following artificial conception feel more guilty than other parents. They should be offered counselling and support from a skilled empathetic person.

*In artificial conception the man masturbates to produce sperms, which is an unnatural act.*

More than 95 per cent of men masturbate. The Biblical injunction against Onan has been perverted. Onan "cast his seed upon the ground" because he did not wish to have intercourse with his brother's widow as Hebrew law enjoined him to do.

*Freezing eggs, pre-embryos and embryos for later replacement is unethical.*

Experience with frozen eggs has shown that the pregnancy outcome is no different from that when fresh eggs are used. There are advantages to the parents if frozen eggs are used. For example, if the first IVF attempt fails, the extra eggs frozen at that attempt can be used for a further attempt without the need for the woman to undergo the invasive procedures needed to obtain eggs from her ovaries.

Freezing pre-embryos and embryos is more difficult, but pregnancies have occurred using a frozen embryo and the technique is improving.

The Royal College of Obstetricians and Gynaecologists reported in 1983 that it was ethical to use frozen eggs and embryos but they added "it would be wise at first to limit the storage time to that required for a foreseeable specific purpose, for example a second pregnancy in the same couple."

In Britain, the Warnock Committee recommended that frozen eggs and embryos should not be stored for a period of longer than 10 years, and the American Fertility Society recommended storage of eggs or embryos for no longer than the "reproductive life of the female donor."

Some women who have achieved a pregnancy may wish to donate some or all of their "surplus" eggs to women who either fail to ovulate or whose ovaries are inaccessible for egg recovery. The ethics of this donation is not different from that of sperm donation for AID.

The disposing of surplus pre-embryos or their use for research purposes raises the ethical question of when human life begins and when the embryo deserves the protection society gives to human beings.

## USE OF EMBRYOS FOR INFERTILITY RESEARCH

*Is it ethical to use eggs and frozen embryos for research, provided the donor has consented?*

The donation of eggs and of very young embryos at an age when the spinal cord has not formed and pain sensation cannot occur would permit the investigation of several problems in infertility that currently cannot be investigated satisfactorily. For example, after a normal conception, about one pregnancy in 10 ends as a miscarriage, and in 60 per cent of them the embryo has not developed normally, the tissues being disorganized and damaged. The use of very young embryos to investigate the errors in cell division might clarify the reason for the miscarriage, and might throw light on the causes of some congenital defects.

There are several other reproductive problems in which donated human embryos might help to improve the "take home baby" rate in artificial conception. At present about 12 per cent of couples entering an IVF program, and about 18 per cent of those who have GIFT or ZIFT, will give birth to a live, mature, healthy baby. If donated embryos were available for carefully regulated research, a higher success rate could be anticipated, since currently, for unknown reasons, relatively few embryos implant in the uterus.

Another area in which research on embryos might improve the results is in cases of defective sperm function. As discussed on page 91 a proportion of cases of infertility are due to the inability of sperm to fertilize the egg. The present methods of investigating defective sperm function, including the sperm penetration test using hamster's eggs, are not accurate. If "spare" human ova were available greater accuracy would probably be obtained and strategies devised to improve the fertilization rate.

These concepts raise moral and ethical problems. A large number of people sincerely believe that the use of human embryos in the research discussed is morally and ethically repugnant, even if it would enable some infertile couples to achieve their desired pregnancy. An equally large number of people approve of the research, provided strict guide-lines were developed and adhered to by the research teams. The extra eggs or very young embryos not required for transfer to the uterus or the Fallopian tubes inevitably die. If they were available for research their contribution to human reproduction could be considerable.

To avoid any possibility of pain, the Warnock Committee recommended that no live embryo be used for research beyond the stage at which the spinal cord is formed, that is 14 days after conception.

*An embryo, although not a human person, is a potential human person and should have the rights of a human person.*

This concept could be construed as applying to sperms and to ova, which are potentially human persons. If it is, it could be considered morally wrong to masturbate, for a male to ejaculate during sleep, to have sexual intercourse at a time when conception cannot occur, for example by using periodic abstinence to avoid a pregnancy. Or is there a difference between a potentially fertilizing sperm or an ovum and a fertilized ovum or an embryo?

*Experimenting on human embryos is morally and ethically wrong as the embryo has a soul.*

The first problem to resolve is to determine when human life begins as compared with biological life. Biological life begins before conception as both the ova and the sperms are very much alive. Human life in theological terms is defined as occurring at the time the soul enters the embryo or the fetus. Some theologians claim that ensoulment occurs at fertilization. This concept raises problems:

1  Many embryos are abnormal due either to chromosome abnormalities or to being defective. Do these embryos have souls?
2  Some embryos divide into two to produce monozygotic (identical) twins. Does the soul divide into two when the embryo cleaves? Or does a second soul enter one or other of the identical twins?
3  In some cases fertilization does not result in an embryo, but in a tumor (trophoblastic tumor or hydatidiform mole), which is potentially lethal to the mother. Does the tumor have a soul?
4  Following fertilization, the fertilized egg divides again and again until it is like a mulberry. At this stage a fluid-filled space appears in it. The inner mass of cells becomes the fetus, the outer becomes the placenta. The two parts are human, have life, but the placenta is discarded at birth. Do only the cells that form the fetus have a soul?
5  If ensoulment does not occur at fertilization, when does it occur? In the past, Christianity and Islam held that the fetus was not a human being until the mother felt it move in her abdomen. This occurs between the 16th and 20th week of pregnancy. In England, for example, in the 18th and 19th centuries a woman could be hanged for murder before the baby had moved in her uterus, but once "quickening" had occurred she was not hanged until she had given birth. In England, even today, a baby stillborn before the 28th week of

pregnancy is not registered as having been born, implying that it has no human identity.

6 A baby born before the 20th week of pregnancy cannot survive outside the uterus. When the gestation period is more than 20 weeks, survival is increasingly possible. In many countries this fact is recognized, and the fetus only becomes an individual after the 20th week of pregnancy.

It seems that it is difficult to determine when ensoulment occurs; it is a theological not a biological concept.

*The new reproductive technologies may lead to undesirable or immoral procedures such as human–monkey hybrids, and cloning.*

These possible, although unlikely, events can be avoided by having strict guide-lines for artificial conception programs. An argument that hybrids might be created is that secretive work by medical scientists may lead to "cloned neo-Hitlers [who] will indeed walk the earth and hybrid hominids [who] will be bred to prey on our own non-processed descendants," to quote an opponent of the new reproductive technologies. The answer is that the integrity of medical scientists, regulated by firm controls approved by the community, will prevent such events. In Britain, the Committee on Artificial Reproduction has approved trans-species fertilization between human and animal gametes as an aid to infertility diagnosis, if it is strictly regulated. A licence to engage in this research is required and issued only if it is agreed that should a hybrid result it would not be allowed to develop beyond the two-cell stage. The sperm penetration test is an example of a human–animal test.

# EMBRYO TRANSPLANTATION

*What are some of the legal and ethical problems associated with embryo transplantation?*

In this technique a donor is artificially inseminated with the semen of the husband of the infertile couple. If a pregnancy results, the embryo is "washed out" of the donor's uterus before it has implanted and is transplanted into the uterus of the infertile wife. The ethical problems of this technique are considerable.

First, does uterine washing out of the embryo place that embryo at undue risk? Opponents of the technology argue that it does as the pregnancy rate following embryo transplantation is low, probably less than 10 per cent. The proponents of the technique argue that as the sterile woman is being given her only chance of having a baby, half of whose genes are those of her husband, and who will be nurtured in her uterus for nearly all of the pregnancy, it is ethically proper to take the chance that the embryo will not survive the transplantation.

A second problem is the question — is the donor "selling" a potential human being, and what are the legal implications for the doctor who engenders the child, by inseminating the donor with the husband's semen, and who washes out the embryo and transplants it into the wife's uterus? Is the doctor encouraging the "sale" of a human being?

A third problem is that the procedure is not entirely safe to the donor. The fertilized egg may implant in a Fallopian tube, causing an ectopic gestation, or the uterine flushing may not expel the embryo. If this occurs the donor has to decide whether to continue with the pregnancy or to seek to obtain an induced abortion.

A fourth problem is to determine to whom the child belongs if the transplantation is successful and a live baby is born. In AID programs, the donor is unknown to the couple, but in embryo donation the donor's identity is known. Further the donor may change her mind and refuse to have the embryo washed out of her uterus. In this case is the husband, who is the genetic father of the child, responsible for supporting the donor and the child after its birth?

Until these legal and clinical problems have been solved, the current (1990) opinion is that embryo donation, obtained by washing out an embryo from the donor's uterus and placing it in the recipient's uterus, should not be performed.

## SURROGATE MOTHERHOOD

*Is surrogate motherhood ethically proper?*

In surrogate motherhood, a woman agrees to be inseminated with the semen of the husband of the infertile couple, and following the birth of the baby, to give the baby to the wife of the infertile couple. The infertile couple agree to pay the surrogate for her services and she, in return, agrees to give the child to the infertile couple.

The legal problems are considerable. First, despite a written contract, the surrogate mother has no legal obligation to give up the child. In law "the person from whose body the child emerges" is the legal mother. Whatever her feelings at the time of conception, she cannot predict before the birth what her feelings about the child will be after the birth and it may cause her great distress to relinquish the baby. Second, the infertile couple may refuse to accept the child if he or she is born with a genetic defect. In this case it is doubtful if the surrogate mother has a legal right to demand that the infertile couple take the child, although she could presumably sue the husband for maintenance. Third, without strict controls surrogate motherhood could be exploited and become a commercial venture.

For these reasons in most countries surrogate motherhood is illegal, although it is undoubtedly occurring.

# WHO SHOULD OBTAIN THE NEW REPRODUCTIVE TECHNOLOGIES?

*The new reproductive technologies should be made available to all couples who choose this way to conceive.*

The argument expressed by some women and men is that today many doctors offer anti-reproductive methods (contraception and abortion) "on demand" or nearly on demand. Why should couples who are pro-reproductive not be given the same choice? To do less, they claim, demonstrates the paternalistic, authoritarian attitude of some of the medical profession. Against this is the fact that the new reproductive technologies are invasive, are costly, the success rate is not high and may be followed by psychological distress in cases of failure.

As was mentioned on page 159, the efficacy of the new reproductive technologies in terms of a healthy "take home" baby is low. If all the menstrual cycles in which the ovaries are stimulated to produce several eggs are taken as the denominator, and the "take home" baby as the enumerator, fewer than 10 babies will result from 100 stimulated menstrual cycles.

It is also evident from published studies that if women with completely blocked Fallopian tubes are excluded, between 12 and 25 per cent of women entering an IVF or similar program will conceive either while on the waiting list or within 2 years of discontinuing the program.

The technologies are expensive. A calculation made in Australia shows that the cost to produce one "take home" baby (which must include the costs of the failures) is at least A$40 000. In addition the costs of operative delivery and the care of the 30 per cent of babies who are premature must be added. The cost is at least twice as high in the USA.

A live healthy "take home" baby achieved by a new reproductive technology is a wonderful gift for an infertile couple, but those infertile couples who fail to achieve this result may not see the technologies in such a light.

From this it is clear that for the community, the costs of the technologies are high. Money spent by the community, that is you and me, through taxes or health insurance, so that a couple may achieve a healthy "take home" baby, must be assessed against the competing demands of money for coronary artery surgery, kidney dialysis, kidney and heart transplants, and the provisions of artificial hips and knees for older people crippled by arthritis.

The health purse is not unlimited and the competing demands for various health care needs has to be discussed much more carefully and widely than at present.

I believe that the new reproductive technologies should only be made available to selected couples who meet strict criteria, and who are attended by trained health professionals working in *licensed* institutions. Those health professionals should be obliged to explain fully what is proposed, the costs and the predictable outcomes, so that the couple can make a balanced assessment of the value to them of the new reproductive technologies.

# 10

## Unexplained Infertility

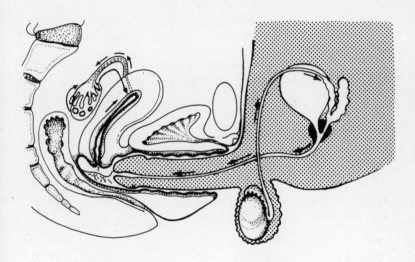

# 10

# Unexplained Infertility

Doctors dislike being unable to make a diagnosis as much, or more, than nature abhors a vacuum. In infertility the dislike is greater because of the distress of an infertile couple who have to be told that even after investigations no reason for their infertility has been found. Unless the couple can be helped to accept this finding, many will start on the sad journey to practitioners of alternative medicine, to orthodox physicians who proclaim a new gimmick and to the numerous charlatans who lie in wait for such a couple.

The criteria that place a couple in the rather unsatisfactory category of unexplained infertility, are shown in Table 10.1.

**Table 10.1   Diagnostic criteria for unexplained infertility**

| | |
|---|---|
| The man | Semen analysis shows normal characteristics<br>? No immunological factors present |
| The woman | Is ovulating regularly<br>Has patent oviducts and no perioviductal adhesions<br>Has no genital tract abnormality, tumor or disease<br>? Has no immunological factors |
| The couple | Have had sexual intercourse at frequent intervals each month for at least 2 years, with intravaginal ejaculation on all or most occasions |

Even these diagnostic criteria cause problems. For example, in recent years the pelvic organs of most infertile women are inspected using a laparoscope. The inspection may reveal fine adhesions that do not distort the oviducts, or tortuous oviducts, or tiny dots of endometriosis. These conditions were not detected before the laparoscope became available. The detection of these minor abnormalities has enabled physicians to classify them as "minor pelvic infection" or "tortuous oviducts," or "mild endometriosis" and thus provide a diagnosis. However, few studies have been made to determine if the treatment of the minor conditions improves the chance of pregnancy. The studies that have been made raise doubts about the value of treatment, as 35–55 per cent of women with minor pelvic infection and between 65 and 75 per cent of women with mild endometriosis become pregnant without any treatment. This is about the same proportion as that of women whose minor pelvic infection or whose mild endometriosis is treated by surgery or drugs. Tortuous oviducts are claimed to be a cause of infertility, but two-thirds of women with this condition (and no other cause) become pregnant within a year when no treatment, apart from the diagnostic laparoscopy and injection of dye through the uterus and oviducts, is given.

Whether these conditions should be included in, or excluded from, the classification of unexplained infertility is unclear. If they are included, unexplained infertility accounts for between 15 and 25 per cent of all couples investigated, whereas if they are excluded the proportion of couples with unexplained infertility is between 10 and 15 per cent. Over a period of 5 years following the infertility investigations 40 per cent of women who have unexplained infertility will become pregnant, whether "treatment" is given or is withheld (Fig. 10.1).

If a couple who, after investigation, are diagnosed as having unexplained infertility, have not achieved a pregnancy within 3

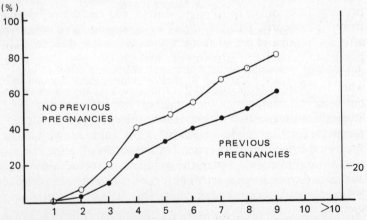

**Figure 10.1**   Unexplained infertility: years before conception

years, IVF or GIFT may be tried. GIFT is followed by a pregnancy rate of about 28 per cent and a "take home" baby rate of about 20 per cent, which is higher than that obtained by IVF. However, GIFT is more invasive than IVF, if the transvaginal pick-up technique is used for IVF, as the sperms and the eggs have to be introduced into the Fallopian tube through a laparoscope.

Women over the age of 35 with a diagnosis of unexplained infertility may have additional problems, as their ovaries respond less well to superovulating drugs. A test has been devised to identify which women are more and which women are less likely to respond. The woman is given the drug clomiphene in a daily dose of 100 milligrams for 5 days. Five days later the level of FSH in her blood is measured. If the level of FSH exceeds 26 milli-international units per milliliter, her ovaries are relatively insensitive and sufficient eggs for IVF or GIFT may not be obtained.

It can be argued that once unexplained infertility is diagnosed and if the woman is aged 35 or over, IVF using the transvaginal pick-up method, or GIFT should be offered without a "waiting period" to see if pregnancy occurs naturally, as women of this age have a lowered fecundity.

## PSYCHOLOGICAL CAUSES FOR INFERTILITY?

It has long been believed that infertility may be due to psychological causes, although there are few well conducted studies to prove or to disprove this belief. Most of the "evidence" derives from case reports, particularly of women who have conceived after adopting a child, or from reports of conception following psycho-therapeutic treatment of infertile couples. Other evidence is slightly more conclusive. In several studies in the past, when the waiting time after the initial investigations were made but before the patency of the tubes was tested was 6 months or longer, it was found that between 10 and 20 per cent of the women became pregnant. Whether the pregnancy occurred because the psychological benefit of deciding to attend the clinic altered hormone levels, permitting ovulation, or altered immunological factors, permitting migration of sperms, or enabled the fertilized ovum more readily to implant in the uterus, remains speculative. Recently a study investigating unexplained infertility reported that of 400 infertile couples investigated by pelvic examination, laparoscopy, investigation of the patency of the oviducts and semen analysis, 16 per cent of the women became pregnant during the investigations and a further 10 per cent became pregnant in the 2 years following the investigations, although no treatment was offered.

The obverse also occurs. It has been observed that a proportion of women who have chosen AID as a means of becoming pregnant temporarily cease to ovulate for the first 2 or 3 months of the treatment, although previously they were ovulating each month.

Current interest in neurotransmitters may offer a clue. It is known that the release from the hypothalamus of gonadotrophin releasing hormone (GnRH) may be inhibited by stress, depression, emotional upsets, anxiety and by certain medications used for the treatment of psychological disturbances. One of the pathways by which the suppression of GnRH seems to be mediated is by increased levels in the brain of opium-like substances called endorphins. Suppression of the pulsatile surges of GnRH will prevent the sequence of events that leads to ovulation, and ovulation may be inhibited. In marked cases the woman will cease to menstruate, but in mild cases she may menstruate although ovulation does not occur. In other cases, the effect may be less obvious and this may be the cause of the few cases of unexplained infertility.

It is also believed that stress may affect the blood supply to the ovaries, leading to a reduction in the quantities of the gonadotrophic hormones reaching the follicles, thus altering the smooth process of ovulation.

Stress-related hormone upset might also affect the function of the oviducts, delaying the movement of the sperms upwards as they seek the ovum, or of the fertilized egg in its passage towards the uterus.

It should be emphasized that these possibilities remain speculative and have not been tested experimentally in humans. Because of the difficulties in human experimentation they may never be tested.

The conclusion remains that at least 15 per cent of couples will be found to have no cause that would account for their inability to conceive a child. When the couple is informed of this, they may feel anger, or grief, guilt or resignation, depending on their personalities. Often, counselling helps (see Chapter 11). A positive statement that offers hope is that without treatment about half of the couples will achieve their desired pregnancy within 5 years. Nevertheless, it is this group of couples who tend to follow the weary pathway of visits to a variety of "experts," who promise that their treatment or surgical technique will produce a pregnancy. These visits are costly in time and money.

# 11

# Psychosocial Problems

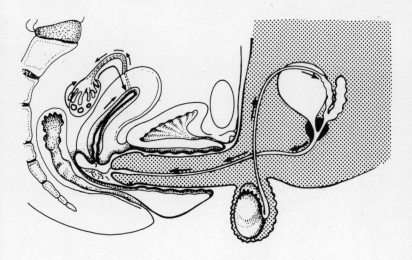

# 11

## Psychosocial Problems

The conception and later the birth of a child is a significant life event. Society expects most of its citizens to marry and, in fact, over 85 per cent do, or if not married legally are in a secure relationship. Within the marriage or the relationship, most couples expect to have children and wish to have children. To most women, motherhood is the expression of her nurturing gender-role and a visible demonstration of her femininity. To most men, fatherhood is the visible evidence of the man's potency and masculinity. To most couples, parenthood is an expression of their love for each other and a demonstration that when they die, their children guarantee that their family survives. To society, childlessness is still regarded as an illness, and by some, as destructive to the community.

If a couple fail to achieve the desired pregnancy, they are seen by many people to have failed their parents and their family, so that their stress may be considerable before they decide to seek help. The woman may see herself as defective, the man may see himself as inadequate, and both may feel guilty as they review their life history to try to detect events they believe might have been responsible for their predicament. For example, a woman brought up in a religious atmosphere may believe that because she had sexual intercourse before marriage, a jealous God is punishing her by rendering her barren. A woman who had an abortion induced at the age of 15 may believe that she is infertile 10 years later, after 2 years of marriage, because of the earlier event. A man whose wife remains barren may attribute her "sterility" to his promiscuity. In the last two examples, the event may have been antecedent of the infertility, but in most instances it is not.

In the 1950s and 1960s a number of psychiatrists believed that more infertile women were psychologically ill than fertile women, and that the psychological stress was a cause of the infertility. Later investigations failed to confirm this hypothesis. The original studies failed to take into account the psychological stress that infertility itself places on the couple, and that this stress may be increased during infertility investigations and subsequent treatment. If the investigations reveal an absolute bar to fertility, or if treatment is not followed by the much desired pregnancy, the psychological upset may become magnified, with considerable emotional strain. This may affect the relationship of the couple adversely, although most couples cope with the disappointment, and their relationship becomes closer, more intimate, rather than more distant.

How can the psychosocial and psychosexual problems be reduced?

1   Investigations that do not have an established value should be kept to the minimum; and older, less informative ones replaced by modern more informative investigations. The fewer the investigations and the less the invasion of each partner's body, the less they feel that the doctor has taken control of their lives. If they feel a loss of control their relationship may suffer and their sex life diminish or become disturbed. The man, expected to have sex on specific pre-ordained days, may lose interest or fail to achieve an erection or may fail to ejaculate. The woman may fail to lubricate and may find penetration painful. Myths, for example that female orgasm or simultaneous orgasm is necessary for conception, may be held, and need to be explored (Table 11.1).

2   The attitude of the doctor who is sensitive enough to note that his patients are victims of their "infertility crisis" may ameliorate the stress. But if the doctor is insensitive and proposes a prolonged series of tests, without explaining their purpose or telling the patients their outcome, their stress may be aggravated. And this in turn, as discussed in Chapter 8, may further reduce the woman's chance of conception.

As I have mentioned, the sequence of investigations should be kept to a minimum, the result of each should be discussed with the couple, and strategies for treatment (if any exist) should be talked about, and other possible tests outlined.

While the investigations are in progress, hope persists, but once a factor causing the infertility has been identified many

**Table 11.1  Infertility myths**

- Masturbation causes infertility
- If you have sex frequently before you marry your chances of getting pregnant are reduced
- Special coital positions increase the chance of conception
- The bigger the woman's breasts the more fertile she is
- Infertile couples enjoy sexual intercourse less than fertile couples
- If a woman is able to relax when she has sexual intercourse she will become pregnant
- Women are infertile because subconsciously they fear pregnancy and motherhood
- Orgasm is necessary for conception to occur

patients (and their partners) go through a number of psychological coping mechanisms. Many couples appear surprised, believing that infertility is uncommon, and that they are isolated by it from their friends, who all seem to have children. The knowledge that between 10 and 15 couples in every 100 are infertile may help them to come to terms with their problem.

Other patients are angry that the intimate investigations required should have been necessary and yet were of no help. Men may believe that the investigations invaded their privacy, forcing them to "have sex at the doctor's demand" or to have to masturbate to produce a specimen, which will be looked at and counted.

Some men, faced with this knowledge, feel that they are no longer masculine, confusing their possible infertility and their sexual response. Others become depressed, sometimes developing erectile failure. The couple may require help to work through these problems.

In other situations, where no cause for the couple's infertility has been discovered, one or other partner (or both) may become depressed as the months, or years, pass and pregnancy fails to occur. Depression, in turn, may inhibit their sexual intercourse or intercourse may be artificially limited to supposed fertile days. The spontaneity of their relationship may go.

Couples who discover, during the course of the investigation, that an absolute or severe barrier to fertility is present may require help. Inability to have children represents a real loss and mourning is an appropriate response. The couple may grieve for their missing child. In their grief, they may seek further opinions, demand further tests, or use exotic treatments in the hope that

pregnancy will result. This is a common reaction in couples
where the investigations fail to disclose any reason for their infertility. And always there is the anecdotal story of a couple who was
given such and such a treatment; or had intercourse in such and
such a position at such and such a time; or ate a specific, if complicated diet; or used this or the other form of exercise — and
became pregnant.

The number of infertile couples, and particularly infertile
women (as they are subjected to more investigations than their
partner), who have these psychological problems is unknown, but
there is no doubt that the "crisis of infertility" is a reality.

In resolving the crisis the doctor and the couple themselves are
involved. The doctor can help to reduce the intensity of the crisis
by treating the problem as a problem of *the couple*, so that neither
is able to "blame" the other. The doctor can limit the psychological upsets inherent in infertility by inviting the couple to undergo
a series of investigations, which are explained, that are sequential
and are discussed. If a particular investigation is of doubtful use,
the couple should have the right to refuse it. Above all the doctor
must be honest in his or her evaluation of the outlook for pregnancy, and should be able to talk comfortably with the couple,
inviting them to talk about their perceived problems, both physical and emotional. It is not enough for a specialist in infertility to
be a good surgical technician, he or she must also be a good
physician and a good communicator. The specialist is perceived
by a couple as important and skilled and may even be invested
with magical powers. What is needed is an expert, but a human
expert.

The doctor must make sure that the couple are given clearly
understood information. Many infertile couples are so anxious
that they do not listen to what is being said. It may help if the
doctor uses a diagram or recommends a book to reinforce the
verbal communication. If the information contains "bad news,"
it should only be given directly to the person or to the couple, not
by telephone. The news often distresses the person considerably,
and if given over the telephone, the distress is increased.

The couple also have a role to play in coping with their infertility. They should try to become well informed and educated
about the problems involved, but should avoid being obses-
sional. They should learn to talk about their problems (if they do
not already do so) so that they can comfortably tell each other
their anxieties, and their fears.

A man who is diagnosed as having azoospermia or untreatable oligospermia during the investigations may experience an enormous blow to his self-esteem and to his sense of masculinity. He may feel inadequate both as a male and a spouse. He may feel he has failed his parents, his wife and society. He may feel he has lost status. Many men equate the ability to father a child with virility. To compensate for being the infertile partner, the man may retreat into depression or compensate by becoming deeply involved in his work, so that he obtains the sense of value denied to him by his "failure" to father a child.

If the investigations show that the woman is the infertile partner, she may also lose her self-esteem. In our society there is considerable pressure for women to bear children. The desire for pregnancy is very strong and the blow to be told that a woman is unlikely or unable to conceive may be devastating. The woman may feel cheated, unfulfilled and deprived, her purpose in life lost. She may go through the phases of surprise, denial, anger, isolation, a feeling of being unworthy, a lack of self-esteem, guilt or grief. The anxieties that may be engendered by these feelings will be reduced if the couple choose to seek counselling or join one of the self-help groups that have been formed so that infertile couples can share their experiences and obtain mutual help in sharing them. Infertility is sufficiently common to make these strategies necessary. As about 15 per cent of all couples are involuntarily infertile, and as only about 50 per cent of them achieve the desired pregnancy, seven couples in every 100 will remain barren, and may need help to adjust to their infertility.

# 12

## The Benefit of
## Treating Infertility?

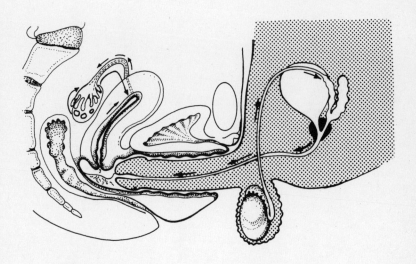

# The Benefit of Treating Infertility?

Two questions need to be asked. The first is "what is the chance of having a live healthy baby after investigation and treatment of infertility?" The second question is "to what extent does treatment help a couple to achieve a pregnancy?"

## SUCCESS RATE AFTER INVESTIGATION AND TREATMENT

In the literature there are reports of several large series of couples who have presented to a doctor with a complaint of infertility. These reports show that in about 90 per cent of cases only one infertility factor can be detected, whereas in the remaining 10 per cent two or more factors are detected. The success rate, in terms of a "take home" baby, will depend on the infertility factor detected, as we have been discussing in this book. There is also evidence that the success rate will depend on the length of time between investigation and conception. For example, some pregnancies occur during investigations, and others occur long after the investigations have been completed.

In 1970 an Australian gynecologist reported that of 503 couples presenting to him with primary infertility, 16 per cent became pregnant following the initial examination of the woman, as did 16 per cent of couples who had secondary infertility. Twelve years later, two Scottish gynecologists reported that 23 per cent of 292 couples with primary infertility and 38 per cent of 108 couples with secondary infertility became pregnant "during or just after investigations."

Since 1980 five large series have been reported, two from Britain, two from the USA and one from Israel. The proportion of couples in which one (or more) of the various infertility factors was detected and the proportion achieving a pregnancy is shown in Table 12.1. The proportion of couples who take home a baby is between 5 and 7 per cent less. The answer to the question: "What is the chance of delivering a live healthy baby after investigation and treatment of infertility?" is that about four couples in every 10 will do so.

**Table 12.1   Pregnancy rates in infertility\***

|  | Proportion of all cases of infertility (%) | Pregnancy rate[†] (%) | Proportion of all pregnancies (%) |
|---|---|---|---|
| *Male:* |  |  |  |
| Azoospermia | 7 | 65 (using AID) | 4.5 |
| Oligospermia | 25 | 30 | 7.5 |
| *Female:* |  |  |  |
| Amenorrhea | 7 | 90 | 6.3 |
| Other ovulatory | 14 | 60 | 7.4 |
| Tubal damage | 16 | 20 | 3.2 |
| Endometriosis (severe) | 2 | 30 | 0.6 |
| Uterine abnormalities | 1 | 70 | 0.7 |
| *Male–female* (Immunological) | 5 | 15 | 0.7 |
| *Unexplained* | 23 | 60 | 13.8 |
|  |  |  | 44.7 |

\*"Take home" baby rates are about 7 per cent lower.
[†]Within 2 years of diagnosis with or without treatment.

The second question: "To what extent does treatment help a couple achieve a pregnancy?" is more difficult to answer. It is unfortunate that the combination of over-enthusiastic doctors and over-demanding infertile couples has prevented the rigorous examination of many tests and treatments. A study made in 1983 by Dr. Collins and his colleagues at Dalhousie University, Nova Scotia, provides some information about this.

Dr. Collins examined the records of 1214 infertile couples his team had investigated between 1 January 1975 and 30 June 1980. Of the 1214 couples, 437 (35.9 per cent) had achieved a pregnancy by July 1981. If the pregnancy had occurred within 3 months of investigation or following medical treatment, or within 12 months of surgery, Dr. Collins believed that the pregnancy was *dependent* on the treatment or surgery. If a longer time had elapsed, or if no treatment or surgery had taken place, Dr. Collins believed that the pregnancy had occurred *independently* of the treatment or surgery. Of the 437 pregnancies, Dr. Collins thought that 171 (40 per cent) were treatment-dependent and 266 (60 per cent) were treatment-independent. He followed up the 1214 couples for longer. Between 2 and 7 years after investigation and treatment, 41 per cent of the treatment-dependent couples, and 35 per cent of the treatment-independent couples had achieved a pregnancy.

He then looked at the pregnancy rate when the couple's infertility problem was placed in one of the categories described in this book. He estimated the percentage of pregnancies occurring in each category and whether each pregnancy was treatment dependent or treatment independent.

Table 12.2 shows that in only three categories was treatment effective in increasing the chance of pregnancy if Dr. Collins' criteria are used. These were amenorrhea of at least 6 months, and usually 12 months, duration; azoospermia treated by AID;

**Table 12.2    Effect of treatment on infertility\***

| Cause | Proportion of total number of infertile patients† (%) | Proportion of pregnancies that were: | |
|---|---|---|---|
| | | treatment dependent (%) | treatment independent (%) |
| Disorders of ovulation: | 28.7 | 51 | 44 |
| Mild or moderate | 26.1 | 50 | 47 |
| Severe | 2.6 | 56 | 22 |
| Male factors: | 28.9 | 35 | 61 |
| Oligospermia | 23.3 | 35 | 75 |
| Azoospermia | 5.6 | 35 | 0 |
| Cervical factor | 4.8 | 46 | 96 |
| Tubal factors: | 15.0 | 24 | 61 |
| Incomplete block | 11.2 | 28 | 68 |
| Complete block | 3.8 | 11 | 0 |
| Endometriosis | 4.0 | 25 | 58 |
| Unexplained infertility | 12.6 | 36 | 96 |

\*41 per cent of the 597 "treated" couples, and 35 per cent of the 617 "untreated" couples achieved a pregnancy.
†Total number = 1214 (from 1983 survey by Dr. Collins of Dalhousie University, Nova Scotia).

and bilateral tubal obstruction treated by surgery. In all other categories similar numbers of pregnancies occurred whether treatment was given or not.

This rather negative report of the value of investigation and treatment of infertility may be too negative. First, the investigations, counselling and reasurance may help the couple dispel their fears and anxiety. Second, since Dr. Collins' report, artificial conception technologies that may reduce the time it takes for a pregnancy to happen, if it is to happen, have been developed. This should reduce the couple's unhappiness. Third, in selected couples the new reproductive technologies will enable a few more couples to achieve a pregnancy and take home a healthy baby (Table 12.3).

### Table 12.3 "Take home" babies as a proportion of women becoming pregnant*

|  | Fertile (%) | Ovulation induced (%) | IVF (%) | GIFT (%) |
|---|---|---|---|---|
| Proportion becoming pregnant | 100 | 70 | 20 | 30 |
| Pregnancy outcome: |  |  |  |  |
| Preclinical pregnancy | 2 | 5 | 10 | 7 |
| Abortion — blighted ovum | 10 | 15 | 15 | 18 |
| Abortion — normal fetus | 2 | 7 | 5 | 5 |
| Ectopic | 0.5 | 5 | 5 | 5 |
| Pregnancy reaching 20 weeks | 85.5 | 68 | 65 | 63 |
| Stillbirths | 1 | 2 | 3 | 4 |
| Proportion babies premature | 8 | 15 | 36 | 34 |
| Proportion multiple pregnancy | 1.2 | 5 | 22 | 22 |
| Proportion of those who become pregnant taking home a baby | 85 | 65 | 59 | 57 |
| Proportion of those entering "program" who take home a baby | 85 | 65 | 12 | 18 |

*Data derived from reports on ovulation induction, and for IVF and GIFT programs, National Perinatal Statistics Unit, IVF and GIFT pregnancies in Australia and New Zealand, Sydney 1988.

Dr. Collins' studies emphasize three important concepts, which should not be lost sight of, either by the couple or the doctor, during the investigation and treatment of infertility:

• First, all proposed investigations should be described to and discussed with the couple before they are made.

• Second, the investigations should be limited to those that have proven helpful. If an unproven investigation is proposed the couple should be told, and the reason why it is being proposed should be explained.

- Third, infertility treatments should be subjected to rigorous clinical trials, before being adopted widely.

# 13
# Unsuccessful Pregnancy

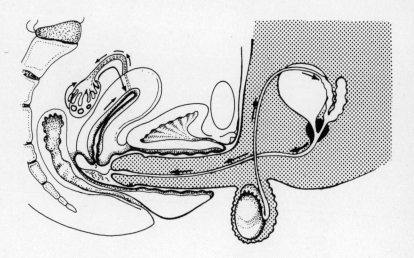

# 13

## Unsuccessful Pregnancy

It has been estimated that following conception a fertile woman has about a 10–15 per cent chance that the pregnancy will terminate in the first 19 weeks of pregnancy. In other words the woman will have an abortion (miscarriage). In addition it is now believed that 20–40 per cent of conceptions may terminate before pregnancy can be diagnosed, in other words, before or during the next menstrual period.

The situation is no different among infertile women who become pregnant, except that the psychological trauma caused by an abortion is greater in many cases.

It is usual to classify spontaneous abortions into two groups: early and late abortions. Early abortions are those occurring before the 10th or 12th week of pregnancy (estimated from the first day of the last menstrual period) and late abortions are those occurring after this time, but before the 20th week of pregnancy. The reason for the division is that the causes of the abortion differ between the two groups, in some cases at least.

## EARLY ABORTIONS

Four-fifths of all spontaneous abortions occur in the first 12 weeks of pregnancy. At least 60 per cent of these abortions occur because the conceptus has chromosomal abnormalities (usually too many or too few) that would prevent it from normal development. In the remaining 40 per cent of cases, it is unusual to find a cause, although many have been postulated. For many years a deficiency in progesterone was believed to cause spontaneous abortion, but careful studies have shown that the reduced secretion of progesterone is a consequence not a cause of an abnormal conceptus.

Infections have been claimed to be a cause, particularly low-grade clinically symptomless infections by such organisms as chlamydia, toxoplasma and cytomegalovirus. Again no real evidence has been obtained. But if a tissue culture obtained from the endometrium reveals certain organisms, in patients who have had three or more repeated abortions, antibiotics may be given in the hope that endometrial infection was the cause of the abortions.

## LATE ABORTIONS

This group accounts for only one-fifth of all spontaneous abortions. In about 5 per cent of cases the cause is a chromosomal abnormality. In some cases the woman's uterus is abnormal, its cavity being distorted by myomata (fibroids) or by an abnormal development. In most cases these conditions would have been detected during the investigation of infertility. The fibroids would have been removed and the uterine abnormality corrected by surgery before pregnancy was attempted. In some cases the woman's cervix is "incompetent." This means that the uterus is unable to contain the growing fetus, and begins to dilate. Incompetent cervix may follow dilatation and curettage, or may be due to a congenital deficiency in its structure. An incompetent cervix is the cause in about 30 per cent of repeated abortions, but is a less common cause of a single spontaneous abortion. If the condition is diagnosed, either clinically or using ultrasound, a "purse-string" suture is placed around the cervix, drawn tight and tied. This simple procedure increases the chance of a woman who has an incompetent cervix giving birth to a live baby from under 30 per cent to over 75 per cent.

Some research workers claim that late abortions (like early abortions) are due to infection by certain bacteria or viruses. These include brucella, chlamydia, listeria, mycoplasma and toxoplasma. The evidence that these organisms cause an abortion is lacking.

Recently a new cause has been postulated, particularly when the abortions are recurrent. This is that there is an immunological problem. The theory is based on the knowledge that the placenta, being derived from the fertilized egg, contains paternal as well as maternal genes, but is not rejected by the mother as foreign. The rejection of foreign tissue is a major problem in transplant procedures, requiring strong immunosuppressant drugs to prevent it occurring. The placenta is partly "foreign" but is not rejected. The reason for this is believed to be that the mother's immune system produces a "blocking" antibody, which covers the antigen sites on the cells of the placenta. This prevents them from being recognized as foreign and rejected.

Scientists who believe that an immunological factor may account for some cases of recurrent abortion claim that if the two parents share similar antigens on their white blood cells (lymphocytes), the mother is unable to make the blocking antibody so that the placenta and fetus are rejected and the pregnancy miscarries. From this, they argue that if the mother is given injections of a donor's lymphocytes before she becomes pregnant again, the foreign lymphocytes will stimulate her immune system to produce blocking antibody. This will coat the antigen sites on the placental cells and prevent an abortion. Recently this concept has been refined. It is now possible to perform a test on the woman's blood that will detect the blocking antibody. If none is found, the injection of donor lymphocytes (or a blood transfusion of concentrated blood) before pregnancy will increase her chance of having a baby the next time she becomes pregnant. On the other hand, if the test shows that she has blocking antibodies, she may have an autoimmune disease (such as systemic lupus erythematosis). In this case corticosteroid drugs may help her to avoid an abortion.

Whether the immune theory of abortion will be sustained requires more research, which must be carefully controlled, or a repetition of the disaster that followed the indiscriminate use of hormones to treat threatened abortion may result.

## THE OUTCOME OF ABORTION

If a woman has a single abortion, her chance of carrying the next pregnancy to the birth of a live healthy baby is excellent. Over 80 per cent of babies conceived after one spontaneous abortion will be born alive and healthy. After two recurrent abortions, 75 per cent of babies conceived will be born alive and healthy; and a similar proportion of babies conceived after three abortions will be born alive and healthy.

## COUNSELLING

An infertile couple need to be aware that they, like any other couple, have a one in 10 chance that the pregnancy will terminate in the first 20 weeks by an abortion. It helps if the couple are able to discuss the problems and receive reassurance that all steps have been taken to reduce this chance by a member of the infertility team.

# Further Reading

1   Behrman, S. J. and Kistner, R. W. (Eds), "Progress in Infertility," 3rd Ed., Boston: Little Brown and Co., 1985.
    A classic textbook. It is rather over-written and long, and propagates some unorthodox opinions, but is a key source of information, provided this is assessed against that of other writers.
2   Harrison, M., "Infertility — a Guide for Couples," Boston: Houghton Mifflin, 1977.
    A "personal" account of her investigations for infertility; dated in the approach and in many of the investigations proposed. Little balance or insight into the problems (although her husband a doctor). Poor on treatment and rather emotional. Easy to read. Good glossary. Others preferred.
3   Hull, M. G. R. (Ed.), "Developments in Infertility Practice" in Clinics, in Obstetrics and Gynecology, 1981, vol. 8 pp. 530–790.
    Written for specialists, this book gives a balanced account of current developments in the field of infertility at the time of its publication in 1981.
4   Kaufman, S. A., "New Hope for Childless Couples," New York: Simon and Schuster, 1980.
    Dr. Kaufman is much aware of the psychological distress caused by infertility and he refers to this in a sensitive way throughout this book. The sequence of investigations is well designed and the chapters on the Basal Temperature Graph and Unsuccessful Pregnancy sensibly and sensitively handled. However, for a book published in 1980, some of the tests described have been abandoned by most infertility specialists and replaced by better, more accurate methods. Examples are Rubin's test and culdoscopy, which have been replaced by the more accurate hysterosalpingography and laparoscopy.
    The book is worth reading and can be recommended.

5   Menning, Barbara, "Infertility: a Guide for the Childless Couple,"
    Englewood Cliffs: Prentice Hall, 1977.
    The author is a nurse specialist in maternal and child health and
    has been unable to become pregnant. She has thought deeply about
    the problem of infertility and this book is the result. The first part,
    "Medical Aspects of Infertility," is poorly presented, unbalanced
    and sometimes wrong. The second part, "Psychosocial Aspects of
    Infertility" is much better and will provide infertile couples with a
    considerable amount of helpful information.
6   Newill, R., "Infertile Marriage," London: Penguin, 1974.
    More factual than Mary Harrison's book, but many of the
    techniques are outmoded (e.g. Rubin's test, testicular biopsy, pro-
    gesterone for threatened abortion) and there are factual errors. Not
    easy to read. The sequence is peculiar and the digressions are often
    irrelevant. At time the contents are directed to specialists in train-
    ing, at times to general practitioners, but most frequently, as
    intended, to infertile couples.
7   Pepperell, R. J., Hudson, B., Wood, C. (Eds), "The Infertile
    Couple," Edinburgh: Churchill–Livingstone 2nd Edition, 1987.
    An excellent textbook, which is written for specialists in infertility,
    but can be read with advantage by family doctors and referred to by
    infertile couples.
8   Stanway, Andrew, "Why Us?" London: Granada, 1980.
    This book contains a considerable amount of useful information
    for infertile couples. It is easy to read and discusses the emotional
    as well as the physical problems associated with infertility, as the
    title suggests. A criticism is that the book tends to give lists of real,
    suspected and possible causes, and is uncritical of some of the
    reported results that are due to chance rather than treatment. There
    are several errors, one major, and some myths continue to be
    propagated in, for example, the section on love-making positions.
    Despite these criticisms the book is recommended.
9   Taymour, M. L., "Infertility," New York: Grune and Stratton,
    1979.
    Although the problems of over-investigation are emphasized and
    condemned, and although the point is made that "the diagnostic
    tests and the therapy involved are as likely to produce emotional
    factors as emotional factors are to produce infertility," the design
    of the book is poor. There is little critical analysis of methods of
    investigation or of treatment, and this diminishes the value of the
    book. The facts are poorly presented and some speculations appear
    as facts.
10  Glass, R. H. and Ericsson, R. J., "Getting Pregnant in the 1980s,"
    London: Univ. Cal. Press, 1982.
    The two authors are respected scientists, one a gynecologist, the

other a research worker in sex-predetermination. Unfortunately, their book is uneven. The main problems that cause infertility are dealt with cursorily, and disproportionate space is given to sex preselection (Dr. Ericcson is Director of a company that claims to help couples preselect their child's sex). Oddly, there is a chapter entitled "Pregnancy after Thirty-five" and one on "Drugs and Pregnancy," which should surely appear in a book on pregnancy, not on getting pregnant. An interesting section of the book is Questions and Answers. Buy the book if you want a transatlantic view.

# Glossary

*Adrenal glands:* two small glands near the kidneys that produce adrenalin, cortisone and small amounts of some sexual hormones

*Agglutination of sperm:* the clumping together of sperm

*Amenorrhea:* the absence of menstruation for a period of 6 months or more

*Amniocentesis:* procedure in which a small amount of amniotic fluid is removed from the uterus of a pregnant woman to examine it for the presence of abnormal cells of the fetus

*Androgen:* generic name for male sexual hormones

*Andrologist:* a specialist in male infertility and male endocrine disorders

*Anorexia nervosa:* an illness resulting from an intense need to avoid becoming fat. The young woman starves herself or else adopts behaviors to help her remain emaciated (see Bulimia). Her weight is less than 20 per cent of the ideal for her height and age and she has amenorrhea

*Anovulation:* the cessation or suspense of ovulation

*Appendicitis:* inflammation of the appendix, usually caused by infection

*Artificial insemination, donor:* the use of an unknown donor's sperm, which is placed in a woman's cervix or uterus to help her become pregnant; known as AID

*Artificial insemination, husband:* the use of the husband's sperm, placed in his wife's cervix to help her become pregnant

*Aspermia (azoospermia):* the absence of any sperm in semen (technically azoospermia means the absence of any *living* sperm in semen, but the terms are used interchangeably)

*Asthenospermia:* decreased motility of sperms

*Biopsy:* a small piece of tissue removed from the body for microscopical examination

*Blastocyst:*   the fertilized egg at the stage of its development when a fluid-filled cavity has formed and cells that will form the embryo can be identified

*Bulimia nervosa:*   illness resulting from a fear of weight gain by women who binge eat and usually use other methods (such as laxative abuse, self-induced vomiting and excessive exercise), to avoid gaining weight

*Cannula:*   a hollow tube

*Capacitation:*   the alteration of the sperm head during its journey through the genital tract, which gives it the capacity to fertilize an ovum

*Cervical polyp:*   benign growth on the cervix

*Cervix:*   lower part or neck of the uterus, which protrudes in the vaginal canal and which contains an opening (or cervix) leading into the uterus

*Chromosome:*   one of the 46 structures that lie inside the nucleus of each cell and carry genes or hereditary characteristics

*Cilia:*   minuscule hairlike forms inside the Fallopian tubes. Their undulant motion apparently helps to push the egg toward the uterus

*Clomiphene*: (brand name Clomid):   a synthetic drug that attempts to stimulate the functioning of the pituitary gland

*Coitus interruptus:*   intercourse in which the male withdraws his penis from the vagina before ejaculation

*Conceptus:*   the embryo or fetus enclosed in the amniotic sac, and the placenta together form the conceptus; all derive from the fertilized egg

*Congenital:*   existing at birth

*Conization:*   surgical procedure in which infected or inflamed parts of the cervix are excised in a cone shape

*Corpus luteum* (Latin for "yellow body"):   yellow mass in the ovary, formed from a follicle that has produced and released an egg. The cells of the corpus luteum secrete progesterone

*Corticosteroids:*   synthetic cortisone-like drugs

*Cortisone:*   hormone produced by the adrenal glands, with many functions relating to many systems of the body

*Curettage:*   the "scraping" of part or all of the lining of the uterus with an instrument called a curette

*Cytoplasm:*   the substance of a cell, which lies outside and surrounds the nucleus

*Dysmenorrhea:*   painful, crampy menstruation

*Dyspareunia:*   pain on intercourse

*Ectopic pregnancy:*   pregnancy that implants outside the uterus, usually in the oviduct

*Embryo:*   developing stage of a fertilized egg from one week after conception to the end of the second month (some define an embryo as an egg from the time of fertilization to the end of the 6th week of its life)

*Endocrine system:* system of glands in men and women including the thymus, pituitary, thyroid, adrenals, testicles and ovaries; the glands produce substances called hormones, which are discharged directly into the blood stream

*Endometrial biopsy:* minor surgical procedure in which a small piece of the endometrium is removed in order to examine it under a microscope

*Endometriosis:* condition in which endometrial-like tissue is present outside the uterus

*Endometrium:* the internal mucous membrane lining the cavity of the uterus

*Epididymis:* oblong structure attached to each testicle where sperm collect on their way to the vas deferens

*Erectile failure:* the inability of a man to achieve or sustain a penile erection (also called impotence)

*Estrogen:* one of the female sex hormones produced primarily by the ovaries in women and, in very small amounts, by the adrenal glands in both men and women

*Fallopian tubes:* two muscular tubes, extending from the upper part of the uterus into the abdominal cavity in which the egg is fertilized, through which it passes from the ovary to the uterus (also called oviducts)

*Fecundity:* the capacity of a woman to become pregnant

*Fern test:* study of dried cervical mucus that can provide presumptive evidence of ovulation

*Fetus:* human developing in the uterus from the end of the second month; known as embryo prior to that stage

*Fibroid tumor:* benign muscular growth, usually in the muscular structure of the uterus; its proper name is a myoma

*Fimbriae:* fringelike outer end of the Fallopian tube

*Fimbriolysis:* surgical procedure in which the fimbriae of the Fallopian tubes are freed from adhesions

*Follicle:* egg sac in the ovary

*Follicle-stimulating hormone (FSH):* hormone secreted by the pituitary gland that stimulates the growth of egg follicles in the female ovary and spermatogenesis in the male testicle

*Gametes:* The male and female reproductive cells, the sperm and the ova capable of entering into union with each other to form an embryo

*Gland:* an organ in the body that produces chemical substances needed for its proper functioning

*Gonadotrophin:* substance capable of stimulating the testicles or ovaries (trophin means growth)

*Gonads:* the sex organs, in other words the ovaries and testicles

*HCG or human chorionic gonadotrophin:* substance extracted from the urine of pregnant women that can be administered by injection to stimulate the gonads. It mostly consists of luteinizing hormone

*Hirsutism:* an obvious growth of hair on areas where hair does not usually grow in women (e.g. the face, the chest, the arms)

*HMG or human menopausal gonadotrophin:* substance extracted from the urine of menopausal women which, when given by injection, is capable of stimulating the growth of ovarian follicles; it consists mostly of FSH; its trade names are Humegon and Pergonal

*Hormones:* substances produced in body glands which enter the blood and produce their effects in other body tissues

*Humegon:* trade name for human menopausal gonadotrophin

*Hydrotubation:* the injection for medical reasons of chemicals or dyes, through the uterus and oviducts

*Hymen:* membrane at the opening of the vagina that partially or fully blocks it

*Hypothalamus:* part of the base of the brain situated above the pituitary gland; it controls activity of the pituitary gland

*Hypothyroidism:* deficiency of the thyroid gland that results in an underproduction of thyroid hormones

*Hysterectomy:* surgical removal of the uterus

*Hysterosalpingography:* X ray study of the uterus and Fallopian tubes, which have been infused with radio-opaque dye to make them visible by X ray

*Implantation:* the embedding of the fertilized egg in the lining (endometrium) of the uterus

*Impotence:* see erectile failure

*Interstitial cells:* (of the testis): see Leydig cells

*Laparoscopy:* surgical procedure in which a telescope-like device is inserted into a woman's abdominal cavity, through an incision in her abdomen, to allow visual examination of the pelvic organs

*Laparotomy:* surgical procedure to explore the abdominal cavity

*Leydig cells:* tiny cells located between the seminiferous tubules in the testicles that are involved in the production of testosterone

*Luteal phase:* second part of a woman's menstrual cycle when a mature egg has been released from the ovary and the corpus luteum has formed and is producing progesterone

*Luteinizing hormone (LH):* hormone secreted by the pituitary gland in women that causes the release of a mature egg from an ovarian follicle and converts the follicle into a corpus luteum

*Meiosis:* the method of cell division of the reproductive cells (the gametes, i.e. the sperms and ova) that results in the number of chromosomes in the nucleus of the cell being reduced by half

*Menopause:* cessation of menstruation that accompanies the end of a female's fertility

*Menstruation:* monthly shedding of the lining of the uterus that occurs in the absence of pregnancy. *Infrequent menstruation* (see oligomenorrhea); absence of menstruation (see amenorrhea)

*Mitosis:* the normal process of cell division; each daughter cell has 48 chromosomes

*Morphology of sperm:* study of the structure and shape of sperms

*Mosaics:* the name given to individuals who have different chromosome complements in different cells. This may result in a physical abnormality or infertility

*Motility of sperm:* ability of sperms to propel themselves forward by means of whiplike motions

*Myomectomy:* surgical excision of myomas (fibroid tumors) of the uterus, leaving the uterus intact

*Necrospermia:* none of the sperm show any motility, i.e. all appear dead

*Oligomenorrhea:* menstrual periods occurring at intervals of more than 6 weeks but less than 6 months

*Oligospermia:* deficiency in the number of sperms in the semen

*Orchitis:* inflammation of the testicle; most commonly caused by mumps

*Ovary:* female sexual gland that produces the eggs and female hormones, located near the uterus and the Fallopian tubes

*Oviduct:* two muscular tubes that stretch out from the upper corners of the uterus towards the ovaries (see also Fallopian tubes)

*Ovulation:* expulsion of a mature egg from a follicle in the ovary

*Ovum* (pl. ova): egg or eggs produced in the female ovary

*Pelvic inflammatory disease* (also known as PID): general name of inflammatory diseases of the pelvis; can be caused by gonorrhea, peritonitis, tuberculosis, or other infections

*Pergonal:* trade-name for Human Menopausal Gonadotrophin

*Peritoneal cavity:* abdominal cavity

*Peritoneum:* membrane lining of the abdominal cavity

*Peritonitis:* inflammation of the membrane lining the abdominal cavity

*Peritubal adhesions:* adhesions of tissue around the Fallopian tubes

*pH:* a measure of the acidity or alkalinity of a fluid. The lower the pH number the more acid the fluid

*Pituitary gland:* gland located at the base of the brain that controls the function of other glands, including the ovaries and testes

*Placebo:* chemically inert substance (usually lactose) used in trials of drugs to test the effect of the mind on the response to treatment. Placebos are also given when no effective treatment is available and the patient wants "something." The word means "I will be pleased" and that is how many people react when given a placebo

*Polycystic ovaries:* formation of multiple cysts in the ovaries, due to an hormonal imbalance

*Postcoital test*: (also known as Sims-Huhner test or the "after intercourse test"): study of a sample of the female cervical mucus several hours after intercourse to determine the presence of sperm, and its ability to penetrate the mucus

*Pre-embryo:* a fertilized egg which has divided once or several times but has not reached the blastocyst stage of development

*Premature ejaculation:* ejaculation of the sperm from the penis prior to or immediately after entering the vagina

*Progesterone:* female hormone, produced by the corpus luteum in the ovary, that helps to stimulate the growth of a uterine lining capable of receiving and nourishing a fertilized egg as well as having other functions

*Prostate gland:* gland located near the bladder and urethra in the male that supplies part of the fluid of the semen

*Psychosomatic:* used to describe physical symptoms caused by or aggravated by psychological or emotional tensions. The symptom is a solution to a problem about which the person is unaware

*Puberty:* age of sexual maturity, when the reproductive organs become functional and begin to release hormones

*Retrograde ejaculation:* condition in men in which sperm are ejaculated into the bladder rather than out through the penis

*Retroverted uterus:* "malpositioned" uterus that is bent backward

*Rubin test:* see tubal insufflation

*Salpingitis:* inflammation or infection of the oviducts

*Salpingogram:* the same as hysterosalpingogram

*Salpingolysis:* surgical procedure to free the oviducts from adhesions

*Salpingoplasty:* surgical procedure to correct blocked oviducts

*Salpingostomy:* another term for fimbriolysis

*Scrotum:* sac that contains the male testicles and accessory organs

*Semen:* liquid produced by the male reproductive organs that contains sperm and other secretions

*Seminiferous tubules:* small twisted tubes in the testicles where sperm are produced

*Sims-Huhner test:* see postcoital test

*Speculum:* instrument that is inserted in the female vagina to allow the visualization of the cervix and the vagina

*Sperm*: (spermatozoon, pl. spermatozoa): male germ cell (or gamete) produced in the testicles, consisting of a small head containing the chromosomes, a neck and a tail

*Spermatogenesis:* production and development of sperm

*Spinnbarkeit:* elasticity of the cervical mucus

*Stein-Leventhal disease:* female syndrome that can have symptoms including infertility, polycystic ovaries, excess hair growth on face and body, and occasionally obesity

*Steroids:*   chemical compounds characterized by a similar "ring" structure. They include most of the sex hormones, cortisone and its derivatives and some other hormones

*Testicle* (Latin, *testis*, pl. *testes*):   male sexual gland, located in the scrotum, where sperms are produced

*Testicular biopsy:*   minor surgical procedure in which a small piece of the testicle is removed to determine if spermatogenesis is taking place

*Testis, testes:*   see testicle

*Testosterone:*   male sexual hormone produced in the testicles and responsible for male sexual characteristics

*Thyroid gland:*   gland located in the neck that produces thyroxine

*Thyroxine:*   hormone produced by the thyroid gland

*Tubal insufflation (Rubin test):*   test in which carbon dioxide gas is passed through the uterus and oviducts to determine if the oviducts are open

*Tubal patency:*   condition in which the Fallopian tubes are unobstructed and open

*Urethra:*   canal to carry urine from the bladder to outside the body; in the male it also carries the seminal ejaculation

*Uterus or womb:*   female reproductive organ, a hollow muscular structure in which the embryo and fetus grow

*Vagina:*   canal between the vulva and the cervix in the woman, into which the male inserts his penis during intercourse. The opening of the vagina is located in the vulva between the urethra and the rectum

*Vaginismus:*   spasm in the muscles surrounding the vagina that prevents intercourse or makes it extremely difficult

*Varicocele:*   dilation of the testicular veins of the spermatic cord

*Varicocelectomy:*   surgical procedure to remove dilated testicular veins

*Vas deferens* (pl. vasa deferentia):   the long muscular tube that conveys sperms from the epididymis to the urethra

*Vasectomy:*   surgical procedure in which a part of the vas deferens is excised

*Vulva:*   the external genitals of a woman

*Wedge resection:*   surgical procedure in which a small section is cut out of the ovary and the ovary is resutured

# Bibliography

This short bibliography gives the reader a chance to find out more information about matters that interest them. Readers should also refer to the two main textbooks about infertility, which have an extensive reference list, mentioned in "Further Reading."

## Chapter 1

Page 19. Relative proportions of the causes of infertility as recently reported in several large series: Katayama, K. P., *Am. J. Obstet. and Gynecol.*, 1970, **135**, 207–12; Templeton, A. A., *Fertil. and Steril.*, 1982, **37**, 175–81; Klinger, B. F., *Fertil. and Steril.* 1984, **41**, 40–46; Hull, M. G. R., *Br. Med. J.*, 1985, **291**, 1643–7.

## Chapter 2

Page 28. Defective luteal phase: Davis, O. K., *Fertil. and Steril.* 1989, **51**, 582–6; Wentz, A. C., *Fertil. and Steril.*, 1982, **37**, 334–6.

Page 39. Use of gonadotrophin releasing hormone: Yen, S. C. C., *Fertil. and Steril.*, 1983, **39**, 257 (a review): Mason, P., *Br. Med. J.*, 1984, **1**, 181; Fauser, B. C., *Fertil. and Steril.*, 1985, **44**, 384–9.

## Chapter 3

Page 56. Genital tract infection in males as a cause of infertility? Naessens, A. (*Fertil. and Steril.*, 1986, **45**, 101) states that screening of seminal fluid for infection is of little practical benefit. Baker, H. W. G., (*Int. J. Androl.*, 1984, **7**, 383–8) says that antibiotics are of little benefit for asymptomatic infection.

Page 56. Prostatic massage of little value in detecting infection (Valvo, *Int. J. Androl.*, 1982, **3**, 104).

Page 58. Varicocele not a cause of low sperm counts: Veermulen, A., *Fertil. and Steril.*, 1984, **42**, 249; Baker, H. W. G., *Br. Med. J.*, 1985, **291**, 1678–80.

Page 62. Problems in evaluating benefits of treatment. See, for example, Bostolfe, E., *Int. J. Androl.*, 1982, **5**, 267.

Page 64. Benefits of clomiphene: Hommonnai, Z. T., *Fertil. and Steril.*, 1988, **44**, 102–5; doubtful: Knuth, U. A., *J. Clin. Endocrinol.*, 1987, **65**, 1081.

Page 65. Adelaide study reported by Kerin, J., *Lancet*, 1984, **1**, 533.

## Chapter 4

Page 77. Optimal time for taking a specimen for the postcoital test. See Taymor, H. C., *Fertil. and Steril.*, 1988, **50**, 702–3.

Page 80. Bristol studies: Hull, M. H. G., *Br. Med. J.*, 1985, **291**, 1693–7.

Page 80. Defective sperm function: Shats, R., *Br. J. Obstet. and Gynaecol.*, 1989, **91**, 37.

## Chapter 5

Page 92. Is the sperm penetration assay of value? See Hull, M. H. G., *Lancet*, 1984, **2**, 245–7; Mao, C., *Am. J. Obstet. and Gynecol.*, 1988, **159**, 279–86.

Page 95. Sex preselection. See Corson, S. L., *Fertil. and Steril.*, 1983, **40**, 384.

## Chapter 6

Page 101. Artificial insemination by donor's sperm. For a review, see Snowdon, R., *The Artificial Family*, Allen and Unwin:

London, 1983; (p. 103) straws given to the woman: McLaughlin, A., *Br. Med. J.*, 1983, **2**, 1110.

Page 105. Intrauterine injection of husband's sperm: No value: Ho, P. K., *Fertil. and Steril.*, 1989, **51**, 682; Glazener, C. M. A., *Br. J. Obstet. and Gynaecol.*, 1984, **94**, 774–8; Wardle, P. G., *Lancet*, 1987, **1**, 270. Some value: Yovich, J. L., *Lancet*, 1986, **2**, 1287.

Page 106. How effective is AID? Hammond, M., *Am. J. Obstet. and Gynecol.*, 1986, **155**, 480–5; Virro, H., *Am. J. Obstet. and Gynecol.*, 1984, **148**, 578.

Page 114. Fresh sperm more effective? Richter, M. A., *Fertil. and Steril.*, 1984, **298**, 277.

## Chapter 7

Page 120. Fibroids distorting uterine cavity indication for surgery: Garcia, C. R., *Fertil. and Steril.*, 1984, **42**, 16–19.

Page 123. Watery or oily contrast medium? DeCherney, A., *Fertil. and Steril.*, 1984, **4**, 698. Higher pregnancy rate if oily medium used: Loy, M., *Fertil. and Steril.*, 1989, **51**, 170.

Page 124. Pain after laparoscopy. See Dobbs, F., *Br. J. Obstet. and Gynaecol.*, 1987, **94**, 266.

Page 132. Hydrotubation no value: Rock, J., *Fertil. and Steril.*, 1984, **42**, 373–6.

Page 133. Pregnancy rates higher after IVF than tubal surgery. See Luber, J., *Am. J. Obstet. and Gynecol.*, 1986, **154**, 1264–70.

Page 133. Table 7.1 based on Donnez, J., *Fertil. and Steril.*, 1986, **46**, 200–4; Luber, K., *Am. J. Obstet. and Gynecol.*, 1986, **154**, 1264; Bateman, B. G., *Fertil. and Steril.*, 1987, **48**, 523–4; Jacobs, L. A., *Fertil. and Steril.*, 1989, **50**, 855–9.

Page 133. "Take home" baby rates low in endometriosis treated by IVF: Wardle, P., *Lancet*, 1985, **2**, 236; *Lancet*, 1986, **1**, 277.

Page 135. Macrophage theory: Holine, T., *Am. J. Obstet. and Gynecol.*, 1983, **145**, 333.

## Chapter 8

The frequency with which publications on the topic of the new reproductive technologies are appearing makes an up-to-date reference list impossible. Interested readers should consult their nearest medical bookshop, or the indexes of the journals *Fertility and Sterility* and the *Journal of In Vitro Fertilization and Embryo Transfer.*

Page 158. The success rate and benefits of the technologies are discussed in several documents and papers. These include: National Perinatal Statistics Unit: *IVF/ GIFT Pregnancies in Australia and New Zealand*, Sydney 1988; Medical Research International: "IVF/ET in the USA in 1985–86," *Fertil. and Steril.*, 1988, **49**, 212–5; Wagner, M., "Are IVF/ET of benefit to all?," *Lancet*, 1989, **2**, 1027–9; Bartels, D., "High failure rates of IVF," *Med. J. Aust.*, 1987, **147**, 474–5.

## Chapter 9

The reader may wish to obtain the various reports from Australia, the UK and the USA, and copies of parliamentary debates in the UK in 1989 and 1990.

## Chapter 11

Lalos, A., *Acta Obstet. Gynaecol. Scand.*, 1985, **64**, 599–604 is a thoughtful paper and provides good references.

## Chapter 12

Collins, J. A., "Treatment dependent pregnancy among infertile couples," *N. Engl. J. Med.*, 1983, **309**, 1206.

## Chapter 13

A good reference book is: M. Bennett and D. K. Edmonds. *Spontaneous and Recurrent Abortion*, Blackwells, Oxford 1986.

# Index